AYURVEDIC BEAUTY CARE

AYURVEDIC BEAUTY CARE

Ageless Techniques
To Invoke Natural Beauty

BY

MELANIE SACHS

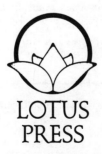

LOTUS
PRESS

Twin Lakes, Wisconsin

DISCLAIMER

If you have an acute or chronic disease, please seek medical attention from a qualified doctor. Although the Ayurvedic principles and practices presented here are beneficial in most cases, they should not be used as a means of clinical diagnosis or treating pathological conditions.

Ayurvedic lifestyle is an excellent adjunct to all forms of medical care, but it is not a substitute for professional care from a physician.

FIRST EDITION, 1994
Printed in the United States of America.

Library of Congress Cataloging in Publication Data:

Sachs, Melanie.
  Ayurvedic beauty care.
  ISBN: 0914955-11X   CIP 93-80313

Published 1994 by Lotus Press/ P.O.Box 325, Twin Lakes, WI 53181 USA

ACKNOWLEDGEMENTS

I would like to send love and gratitude to:
My teachers . . .
Dr. David Frawley
Margo Gal
Dr. Shalmali Joshi
Dr. Sunil Joshi
Dr. Vasant Lad
Amadea Morningstar
Dr. Pankaj Naram
Dr. Smita Naram
Dr. Lobsang Rapgay
Dr. Robert Svoboda

To those who encouraged me to formulate this book . . .
Ella Helgrin
Marilyn Hunt
Mrs. Neeta Kale
Rex Lassalle
Elizabeth Ray
Dorothy Parks
Jo Wackett

To those who helped make my first booklet, *"Invoking Beauty with Ayurveda"* . . .
Susie Biggs—computer work
Morag Charlton—graphics, layout, and model
Karuna Fluhart—photographer

Bob Sachs—editor
Dianna Shannon and Rita Zamora—models

Friends who worked on this book with quality and care . . .
Thomas Bonner—photography
Morag Charlton—graphics
Barbara Falconer—cover art & design
Bob Sachs—typing and provisional editing
Lenny Blank, Margie Hughes, Connie Durand, Buffalo
Publications, Lavon Alt and Santosh Krinsky

To the beautiful friends who volunteered as models . . .
Valencia Dela Vega
Ann Levin
Carol Merrill
Ashley & Shelly Miller
Peggy Moor
Kai Ling Sachs
Victoria Tieje

Friends who took the time to write testimonials . . .
Deb Bergeron
Dave Davenport
Patricia Deva
Karuna Fluhart
Michelle Herman
Carol Hoy
Wendy Portman
Margaret Thompson
Detchen Wallace

To my family—my husband Bob, and my children, Kai Ling,
Christina and Jabeth, for helping me take the time to write . . .
And to my beloved family in England for all their kindness and
support, always.

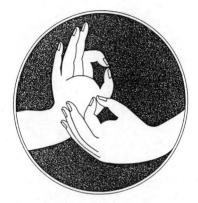

DEDICATION

This book is dedicated
with love
to my parents,
Penny and Percy Brown,
who taught me to treasure and respect
the beauty of nature
and
the power of the human
spirit.

CONTENTS

FOREWORD

On the eve of entering a long period of silence on the banks of the Ganges River with the wise and the ancient, I find resounding joy to applaud Melanie Sachs in her present effort on Ayurveda. Three years ago I introduced the Ayurvedic concept of beauty in *Diet for Natural Beauty*. When a colleague, Bob Sachs, asked me if I would consider writing the Foreword for his wife, Melanie's, book, *Ayurvedic Beauty Care*, I reflected on the miracles of providence.

The sages of beginningless time gave a legacy to the universe. It carried the secret codes of the divine plan. Ayurveda holds these secrets of health so excellent, that in the knowing, the human body may illuminate as a crystal reflecting the infinite. "Rasa" is our essential nature and the secret code which guides our choices. It is the beauty of the universe which we reflect. Rasa is in every grain of sand and every morsel on which we feed. It keeps our intentions sacred. Deep within our cognate nature, we have the memory of all time embedded in us. Our potential to know this beauty of self is as infinite as our timeless memories. It is only through inquiry and knowing of our real nature that we are able to own this energy of numinous joy.

Melanie brings a fresh and unique perspective to the practice of this ancient body of health and beauty care. Her simple offering on the body types, the cleansing therapies, and the immortal aesthetics of Ayurveda makes this an easy-to-use manual.

Melanie has been refining her life of healing for a long time. Through Ayurvedic practices she was able to heal herself from the deep pain of losing a child, and later from cervical cancer. In this book she has culled a rich variety of information and sadhanas from her personal practice in Ayurveda, and from her life as both teacher and mother.

Ayurvedic Beauty Care is a reverent work, celebrating the fineness of the human spirit which has claimed its light. This offering reaches everyone who is interested to learn and share these ancient secrets of excellent health.

Bri Maya Tawari

Asheville, N.C.
December 9, 1993

INTRODUCTION

Ayurveda was revealed to the seers of India thousands of years ago. In a natural environment supportive of all life, these seers or "rishis" came to understand the principles by which health and well-being is both created and destroyed. Ayurveda, the "science of longevity," promotes positive health, natural beauty, and long life. This science was first recorded around 2500 years ago. Although rooted in antiquity, Ayurveda is based on universal principles and is a living, growing body of knowledge—as useful today as it was in centuries past.

Traditional Ayurveda fits quite well into modern models of holistic healing, concerned with a broad view of the total health of the individual: physically, emotionally, and spiritually. What Ayurveda offers to these models beyond its own techniques is a deeper awareness of how the body and our experiences are a microcosm of the greater universe and the relationships in the interaction between our inner and outer worlds.

Ayurveda teaches that health is maintained by the balance of three subtle energies, known as Vata, Pitta, and Kapha. These energies account for all forms of matter (Kapha), the force and direction they move (Vata), and the transformations they go through (Pitta). As all life forms possess these qualities, the purpose of Ayurveda is to bring these forces into harmony so that they promote physical, emotional, and spiritual growth. All Ayurvedic treatments are designed to return these forces to an harmonious balance rather than concentrate on what their imbalance manifests. Thus it focuses on causes rather than symptoms. And as each individual has their own particular balance or blend of these three forces, Ayurvedic treatments are person, rather than disorder, specific. Such an approach has proven effective over the centuries and as a result, many of Ayurveda's healing regimens have been adopted and refined by peoples all over the world. This may be the reason why it is considered the "mother of all medicines."

While Ayurveda has included in its body of knowledge the use of surgery and powerful medications, it also has intact systems of daily health care practices: diet, exercise, meditation, herbology, and rejuvenation therapy. Such practices are not just palliative. They are considered an integral and respected part of the healing process. Many of these practices have found their way into the practices of Western healers who have adapted them to the demands of western culture and a changed global ecology. As such adaptions are in keeping with Ayurvedic principles, they should be honored for their contribution to the advancement of Ayurveda into the 20th century. This demonstrates the vitality and adaptability of the "mother of medicines."

The Role of Beauty in Ayurveda

When we talk about beauty in the context of Ayurveda, it should be perfectly clear from the start that we are not talking about market-driven ideals of the moment. In Ayurveda, inner and outer beauty are intimately related. The more we nurture ourselves, the more radiant we become physically and expressively—regardless of our particular body shape or proportions.

In keeping with the general orientation of eastern philosophy and healing, beauty can be viewed as having three aspects; an outer, inner, and secret aspect. When one balances the outer and inner, one has accomplished the secret aspect.

Outer beauty is what we most commonly associate with the field of beauty. It is the perfection of what is visually perceived. It includes the obvious traits such as contours of the body, texture of the skin, and the quality of the hair and nails. But in Ayurveda it also includes grace in posture and movement and the subtle qualities of freshness and vitality and magnetizing brightness of being. Like today's authorities on natural body care, Ayurveda has always understood beauty to be the product of general physical health and appropriate daily care. It is not just a cosmetic event. The emphasis is on self-knowledge and development of positive routines and habits that literally will bring out the best in ourselves. It makes true good looks possible. Even as we grow older, with appropriate care, we will mature with a strength and vitality which will bring out a new depth to our outer beauty—a beauty born of life experience.

Inner beauty relates to inner qualities of being, including emotional states and mental abilities. Like physical qualities, they are largely determined at birth and are considered to be the result of actions and aspirations from previous lives. As physical form can be molded by diet and lifestyle, we can also train our minds to cultivate positive states of being. Just as the body can be purified and strengthened to make it outwardly more beautiful, so the mind can become tamed and disciplined. The start of this process is to begin to accept who we are and begin to truly care for and appreciate ourselves. With mind training, the ability to relax while concentrating helps us to be alert and more aware in the moment. This moves our whole being naturally towards our greatest human potentials and activities—to act skillfully in the world with compassion and loving kindness.

The secret aspect of beauty refers to the energy, insight, and inspiration it takes to balance the inner and outer. Developing this special quality takes time, patience, and a willingness to learn from experience. This is the mark of real maturity that ripens into deep lasting beauty that is experienced from within and seen by all from without.

As Maya Tiwari so beautifully put it in her contribution to *Diet and Beauty* (Japan Publishing), "The three aspects of beauty are like a scale, one side holds the *alankaras,* or external ingredients, while the other hold the *gunas,* or internal ingredients. And the act of balancing itself is the third aspect, or *rasa.* . . . This is magic. This is maturity. And this is beauty in its fullness."

In this spirit, I present here both ancient and modern Ayurvedic secrets for beauty care and enhancement. The aim is to elevate our western understanding of beauty to new levels with the deeper Ayurvedic insights. These insights hold powerful health promoting and enhancing methods and luxurious beauty techniques such that all levels of beauty (outer, inner, and secret) can be realized in our increasingly fast-paced and chaotic world.

There are two audiences that I address in this volume. First and foremost I want every person to be able to find what brings out their true beauty. In this light, the book is intended to be a self-care manual. At the same time, I want all those interested in or practicing as beauty therapists or aestheticians to receive the benefits of the deep insights and marvelous results Ayurveda can offer their clients.

How to Use this Book . . .

1) Start by discovering your "prakruti"—the unique blend of universal energies that came together to give you both your body type and temperament.

2) Next, read on to understand a little more about the Ayurvedic view of how the body is nourished in the chapter on Dhatus. Together, these two steps give you the background and encouragement for making lifestyle choices that will bring out your inherent strengths and natural beauty described in subsequent chapters.

As health supports beauty, guidelines for appropriate lifestyle choices will always be an equal partner with the more specific beauty care techniques in producing natural beauty. Though these health care choices are not essential to the immediate effectiveness or enjoyment of using Ayurvedic beauty care, they definitely enhance the results, especially over the long term, and will help to address and ameliorate long standing complaints. Of the lifestyle factors that will be discussed, the two that are most emphasized are diet and massage. Diet nourishes all the body tissues creating healthy muscle tone, clear skin, and a natural aura of well-being. Massage works on all levels, improving the complexion, skin tone, body posture as well as nourishing the inner self.

3) Select exercise regimens, relaxation techniques and daily beauty care practices that are suited to your "prakruti."

4) People wishing to nurture partners and for beauty therapists and aestheticians, the chapter on the Ayurvedic Facial Sequence will stand out on its own as a unique, nurturing, and beneficial beauty care practice.

5) Read about and take the opportunity to experience the special Ayurvedic treatments.

6) *Enjoy the results.*

WHAT IS YOUR PRAKRUTI?

Prakruti literally means "the first creation." It is determined at the point of conception and refers to the innermost nature of an individual. It is the unique blend of qualities that makes each of us, from the point of conception, completely unique. We are individually formed yet are still an integrated part of the universe from which we were born. Discovering your Prakruti is the beginning of understanding the qualities of your uniqueness. Becoming familiar with these qualities is your guide to knowing how to best take care of yourself and bring forth your own unique, natural beauty.

To better understand prakruti you must first understand how Ayurveda views the body. Individuals are considered to take form as a result of three life-giving forces. These forces are called *"doshas,"* namely *Vata, Pitta,* and *Kapha.* They are considered simply as the inherent intelligence of the body: they are the invisible forces that orchestrate all the functions of the body, thus shaping how we look, how our metabolic processes function, how we respond to different surroundings, even how we think and feel.

For example, it is the influence of Kapha that makes us salivate when we are hungry and see something that we want to eat. It is Vata that facilitates swallowing the food and Pitta that makes the digestion process possible. In this way we can see that it is vital that doshas work together in harmony for the body to work to its maximum potential. Likewise the imbalance of the doshas is viewed in Ayurveda as the underlying cause of all physical, mental, and spiritual problems.

The physical body is considered to be a combination of two kinds of substances:

• retainable substances or substances that stay as part of the body

1

known as "*dhatus.*" These are what we commonly know as plasma (*rasa*), blood (*raka*), muscle (*mamsa*), fat (*meda*), bone (*asthi*), bone marrow (*majja*), nerve and reproductive tissues (*shukra*).

• unretainable substances, that is, substances that leave the body, known as "*malas.*" These are the waste products of the body; fecal matter, urine, sweat.

Then we have *Agni,* the ruler of all the metabolic processes. Agni is the transformer of what is outside to that which we take in and becomes part of our body or recorded experience. For example, while it is Agni that digests food in the stomach so tissues can be built, it is also, less obviously, agni in the mind that digests experiences to form impressions and memories.

Bringing balance and health to the whole system (doshas, dhatus, malas, and agni) is the fundamental principle of Ayurvedic healing. It is also how Ayruveda engages the body to bring forth its own inherent individual beauty.

This chapter will focus on the doshas and the qualities they bring to the body.

The Doshas

The doshas are themselves combinations of energy we name the Five Elements.

EARTH—the solid state of matter.

WATER—the fluid state of matter.

FIRE—the energy or power to transform matter from one state to another.

AIR— the gaseous state of matter.

ETHER—the space in which matter can exist and is contained.

The three doshas are the manifestations of these five states in the body.

Vata is a combination of AIR and ETHER. It is responsible for all movements of the body, mind, and senses and the process of elimination.

Pitta is a combination of FIRE and WATER. It is responsible for heat, metabolism, and energy production and digestive functions of the body.

Kapha is a combination of EARTH and WATER. It is responsible for physical stability, proper body structure, and fluid balance.

Each of the doshas has characteristics that manifest in the body and mind as particular qualities. These qualities are what you might expect from the characteristics of the associated elements.

VATA	PITTA	KAPHA
dry	oily	oily
cold	hot	cold
light	light	heavy
irregular	intense	stable
mobile	fluid	viscous
rarefied	acidic	dense
rough	liquid	smooth
quick	sharp	dull

The unique characteristic of Vata is dryness, Pitta heat, and Kapha, heaviness. So, we say that whenever there is a lot of dryness in the body, Vata energy is high. This may be dry skin, dry hair, cracked lips, or internal dryness resulting in constipation. When there is excess heat, Pitta energy is high, as in the case of fevers and inflammations, or hot temper. When there is excessive heaviness, extra Kapha energy is present, making for excess weight, cellulite, water retention, swelling, or puffiness.

Your prakruti does not change; it remains constant throughout life. The state of the doshas can change. This changed pattern is called *vikruti* or conditional state, as it does not match the original pattern. It causes disruptions that eventually result in some kind of disorder. Let's examine a little closer at how this vikruti comes about.

The attributes given to Vata, Pitta, and Kapha exist all around us. They manifest in the climate, living conditions, emotional atmosphere, and in the foods we eat. These qualities from our environment act on our bodies, bringing to it their qualities. The outer elements are directly changing the balance of inner elements.

For example:

Wind, being drying in nature, increases Vata dosha causing the skin to become dry and cracked.

Greasy, spicy foods, being heating and oily in nature, increase Pitta dosha which can cause oily or acne skin.

Excessive sleep, being Kapha in nature, increases Kapha dosha. This inertia contributes to weight gain.

This is known as the principle of like increasing like. By the same logic, influences of opposite qualities to the dosha will help to maintain balance. These are fundamental principles of healing in Ayurveda and the key to making correct choices to support the health and beauty of the body.

For example:

Vata is cold and spacious, so it is useful for those of high Vata nature to keep warm at all times. Internal cold, balanced by external warmth, relaxes the body and is grounding.

Pitta is hot and oily so it is wise for high Pitta-types to be conservative with their consumption of greasy foods. In addition, choosing spices, herbs and condiments that have a cooling effect and help with the digestion of fat is useful.

Kapha is dull so it is useful to keep high kapha types mentally stimulated and physically active.

This view of the nature of life is not meant to be another convenient way to categorize people. Nor is there any judgement as to which mixture of doshas is better than the others. One combination of energy is never inherently better than another. Each has its own potential vices and virtues and ability to be in balance or not. Discovering your prakruti should be viewed as an opportunity to better understand your own individuality. Becoming familiar with your given energy network, living it, and learning to keep it in harmony is basic to Ayurvedic beauty care, as well as having a long, rich and happy life. Everyone can be beautiful in their own way.

Please remember that your Prakruti or individual dosha balance is classically determined by the highly developed skill of taking of the pulse. As many readers may not have access to a good pulse diagnostician, the following charts are provided to give just some indication of your dosha balance. This is practical from the beauty care point of view, as you are aiming to tame symptoms. For truely assessing prakruti, they are not conclusive. Please do not use them to draw firm conclusions, but rather as a means to raise awareness of your own nature and that of others, honoring physical differences and ways of approaching life. Becoming aware of and communicating well with your body, together with the simple Ayurvedic guidelines presented here, is all you need to help yourself towards lasting grace and beauty.

On Identifying Attributes . . .

When identifying attributes that are most like your own (or whoever you are classifying), compare to those who share the same ethnic and racial background.

Next to each attribute you will find a blank line. For your easy reference, check attributes as you identify with them. Sometimes more than one attribute will be found on a given line. In that case, if you identify with at least one of the attributes on that line, check for the entire line.

VATA: Body Type
_____ slender in build or overweight
_____ thin as a child
_____ under-developed muscles, flat chest
_____ fine, small bones and/or prominent joints
_____ unusually tall or short in height
_____ Narrow hips and shoulders or narrow hips and wide shoulders or visa versa

_____ limbs and fingers and toes are stubby or long and slender

_____ joints tend to crack, pop, ache, or strain easily

_____ tend to put weight on at the midriff; weight is hard to gain and relatively easy to lose

_____ veins and tendons are prominent, especially in hands and chests

_____ small breasted or disproportionately large breasted

_____ darker complexion or light, but sallow or with a grayish cast; tans easily and deeply without burning

_____ skin cold to touch, dry and rough, especially hands and feet

_____ skin is thin and fine pored; sometimes dry in patches

_____ few moles that are dark in color

_____ skin problems with dryness, especially in winter; other conditions may include psoriasis, dry eczema, leathery texture, corns, calluses, cracks

_____ body hair either scant or overabundant; dark, coarse and curly or very fine

_____ head hair tends to be dark, coarse, wiry, kinky, frizzy

_____ hair tangles easily, prone to be dull with split ends, dry and oily areas, dandruff

_____ nails are hard, brittle, variable in shape and size; sometimes ridgy, bitten with hangnails, and have pale bluish cast

_____ eyes are grey, violet, slate blue, or dark chocolatey brown in color

_____ eyes unusually large or small, or different in size, irregular in position, dry, with bluish whites

_____ eyes dart around or twitch; can be itchy

_____ eye lashes are short, scanty, dry, or extra long

_____ eyebrows are thin

_____ mouth large or small with large, thin, or unbalanced top and bottom lip _____teeth irregular in size, tendency to protrude, brittle, prone to gum recession

_____tongue often heavily coated with a thin grayish pink coating

_____lips dry, prone to cracking, especially in winter

_____nose thin, small nostrils and often deviated septum

_____ears thin, bony, and irregular in shape; small lobes

_____gait is quick and light

_____digestion changeable; can have gas, constipation, sometimes diarrhea

MENSES

_____cycle irregular

_____longer between periods

_____scanty, clotty flow

_____dark blood

_____accompanied by constipation and severe cramps

APPETITE

_____varies

_____eyes bigger than stomach

_____loves crunchy snacks

_____needs to eat frequently

_____becomes very weak with fasting

CRAVINGS

_____dry, crunchy snacks

_____salty, sour foods

_____eating a lot or very little

SEX DRIVE

_____appetite varies

_____very passionate

_____tires easily

_____has many fantasies

_____low fertility

ACTIVITY
_____ very restless
_____ low stamina
_____ tends to be over-enthusiastic and then overdo
_____ poor body tone and coordination
_____ hungry after exertion
_____ rarely sweats
SLEEP
_____ either light or very deep
_____ hard to get off to sleep because of active mind
_____ sleep often broken
_____ rarely feels well rested
_____ grinds teeth
_____ sleep walk
DREAMS
_____ active, violent, intense, vivid
_____ many, but often forgotten
_____ of being chased or flying
VOICE
_____ hoarse, cracky, breathy
SPEECH
_____ fast speaking and very talkative
_____ strays from subject, long winded
_____ enjoys monologues
_____ talks to anyone or anything
MOVEMENT
_____ quick and darting
_____ weak and light
CLIMATE
_____ loves sun and warmth
_____ miserable, nervous in high wind, dryness, and cold
_____ benefits by being in quiet, wide open spaces

FINANCES
____ spends freely
____ buys in quantity on whim
LIFESTYLE
____ difficulty in creating useful habits
____ living space very full and/or untidy
MEMORY
____ variable
____ better at short term than long term
____ quickly can forgive and forget
THINKING STYLE
____ loves to theorize, very flexible, brain stormers
____ not interested in practical application
____ thinks in words
____ don't make decisions easily
SENSITIVE to
____ noise, pain, cold, drafts
UNDER STRESS, experiences
____ fear, anxiety
____ excitable
EMOTIONS
____ emotional and changeable for no particular reason
____ creative, alert, active, restless
____ weak willed; easily knocked off center

PITTA: Body Type
____ medium in build
____ medium build as child
____ athletic musculature
____ medium bone structure
____ average in height
____ medium hips and shoulders that are well proportioned
____ well proportioned limbs, hands, and feet
____ joints normal; not a problem

_____ put on weight evenly; can be willfully successful at losing weight

_____ veins and tendons moderately prominent

_____ medium breasted

_____ normal or slightly oily, fair, coppery, or pinkish complexion; freckles and burns easily

_____ skin is warm to the touch all over

_____ delicate skin prone to premature wrinkles, oily in the "T" zone; inflammation and itchiness; blushes easily

_____ many moles and freckles that are bluish or brownish red

_____ skin problems may include rashes, acne, blackheads, whiteheads, dry and oily areas, reddish-brown blotches

_____ body hair light and fine

_____ head hair is red, blonde, light, prematurely grey, fine, silky; balds prematurely

_____ hair gets oily quickly, especially in hot weather which dulls the hair

_____ nails are rubbery yet strong, even oval shape, with a pink, coppery cast

_____ eyes hazel, green, light blue, electric blue

_____ eyes medium in size and evenly placed; sun and chemical sensitive and with fine red lines in the whites

_____ average eyelashes and eyebrows

_____ eyes sharp, alert, direct, penetrating

_____ mouth medium in size with even lips

_____ teeth even, yellowish; prone to cavities and bleeding gums

_____ tongue occasionally coated with yellowish, orange, red film; may experience sores in mouth

_____ lips prone to cold sores

_____ nose medium in size, prone to thread veins

_____ ears medium in thickness, even in shape, with medium lobes; may be red and warm

_____ strong digestion; upset by large volumes of hot, spicy, or greasy foods

MENSES
_____ cycle regular
_____ bleed for longer period
_____ intense flow
_____ bright red blood
_____ accompanied by loose bowels and mild cramping

APPETITE
_____ strong
_____ greatly enjoys food; social eaters
_____ likes spicy, hot, and oily foods
_____ irritable if miss or late for meals
_____ does not like to fast

CRAVINGS
_____ greasy foods
_____ spicy foods
_____ iced drinks and cold foods

SEX DRIVE
_____ strong desire
_____ passion well controlled
_____ average stamina
_____ anger if desires not fulfilled
_____ average fertility

ACTIVITY
_____ very efficient, precise, and orderly
_____ compulsive, competitive
_____ average stamina, except in heat
_____ exhausted by overeating
_____ good tone and coordination
_____ hungry and thirsty after work
_____ sweats easily; tendency for strong body odor

SLEEP
_____ sleeps lightly

_____ easily gets to sleep unless worried

_____ rarely broken

_____ feels alert, even after many nights of light sleep

_____ troubled if worried by work issues

_____ night sweats

DREAMS

_____ passionate, colorful

_____ remembered well

_____ dreams of chasing, competing, buying, selling

VOICE

_____ intense, piercing, clear

SPEECH

_____ impatient tone, well measured

_____ sharp tongued, precise

_____ loves to debate

_____ talk to anyone they feel are intellectual equals

MOVEMENT

_____ direct, precise, and assertive

CLIMATE

_____ loves cool weather

_____ irritable in heat and high humidity

_____ benefits by being near clear lakes, oceans, rivers

FINANCES

_____ efficiently manages money

_____ spends on top-of-the-line items

LIFESTYLE

_____ well organized

MEMORY

_____ reasonable

THINKING STYLE

_____ planners, visionaries, organizers

_____ like to find practical applications

_____ think in pictures

SENSITIVE to
_____ heat, light, color
UNDER STRESS, experiences
_____ anger and irritability
MIND
_____ intelligent, ambitious
_____ strong, forceful, stubborn, determined
_____ critical
_____ perceptive, joyous, confident
_____ perfectionist
_____ pride
_____ idealistic, enterprising, intense
_____ vain
_____ revengeful
_____ jealous
_____ self-centered

KAPHA: Body Type
_____ heavy in build; large, strong, stable
_____ plump or chunky as a child
_____ thick musculature
_____ heavy bone structure, but not prominent
_____ medium in height
_____ broad frame, especially at hips and shoulders
_____ well proportioned limbs
_____ joints move very smoothly and freely; well lubricated
_____ put on weight around the bottom and hips; weight is
         easily gained and lost with difficulty
_____ veins and tendons well covered by thick skin
_____ heavy breasted
_____ pale skin that burns after long exposure to sun; tans
         evenly after moderate sunbathing
_____ skin cool to touch but rarely have especially cold hand or

_____ feet
_____ skin has pale, gleaming white tone, soft, moist, thick, smooth, slightly oily and tendency towards large pores
_____ few moles, may have white or tan blotches
_____ skin problems are rare, but may include skin sensitivity, large open pores, pustular acne only in extreme cases
_____ moderate amounts of heavier body hair
_____ head hair is dark or light; thick, heavy, wavy
_____ though only slightly oily, hair is lustrous
_____ nails are strong, thick, large, square, symmetrical, and pale in color
_____ eyes are milk-chocolatey brown
_____ eyes are large, liquidy, tranquil
_____ eyelashes and eyebrows are thick and heavy
_____ eyes look steady and calm
_____ mouth is medium with full, even lips
_____ teeth large, even, gleaming white and strong
_____ tongue, if coated, has thick, white, sometimes greenish and curd-like coating
_____ lips are moist
_____ wide nose with large nostrils
_____ ears are thick, even shaped with large lobes
_____ digestion is steady; can get sluggish

MENSES
_____ regular
_____ effortless
_____ average flow
_____ light colored
_____ dull, mild cramping with water retention

APPETITE
_____ stable
_____ emotional eaters
_____ loves sweet, starchy foods

_____ missing meals is not a problem
_____ can most benefit from fasting
CRAVINGS
_____ sweet, sticky desserts
_____ smooth, creamy textures
SEX DRIVE
_____ steady desire
_____ once inspired, deeply involved
_____ great stamina
_____ very intense and strongly attached
_____ very fertile
ACTIVITY
_____ prefers to be still
_____ enduring stamina if inspired
_____ greatly benefits from exercise
_____ slow and methodical
_____ good tone and coordination
_____ little hunger or thirst after work
SLEEP
_____ deep and for long periods
_____ easily sleeps, even in daytime
_____ rarely broken
_____ sluggish in morning; needs 8 hours at least
_____ feels rested and refreshed by sleep
_____ snores
DREAMS
_____ cool, peaceful, uneventful
_____ rarely forgotten, but of little consequence
_____ pastoral scenes, strong emotional content
VOICE
_____ gentle, sweet, melodious
SPEECH
_____ slow, deliberate

_____ few words
_____ kind, loving, encouraging words
_____ will not speak until spoken to
MOVEMENT
_____ slow and flowing, relaxed
CLIMATE
_____ loves warmth, sunshine, and comfort
_____ suffers in high humidity, cold and damp
_____ not strongly effected by weather changes
FINANCES
_____ saves and stewards wealth well
_____ spends emotionally
LIFESTYLE
_____ habitual
MEMORY
_____ slow to learn, contemplates deeply
_____ very good once information has sunk in
_____ holds onto old hurts
THINKING STYLE
_____ stable, but flexible
_____ reliable and trustworthy for running operations
_____ thinks in concrete terms
SENSITIVE to
_____ touch and emotions
UNDER STRESS, experiences
_____ (is generally stable, but if pushed to extreme) fear and anger
MIND
_____ tolerant
_____ courageous
_____ calm, placid
_____ generous
_____ dullness, depression, heaviness, narrow minded, loyal to
        friends

_____ understanding
_____ greed
_____ attachment
_____ envy
_____ possessive

OVERVIEW OF THE THREE DOSHAS

Once you've gone through the above lists, use the following lists as a summation of key characteristics. Keep these points in mind to better understand the Ayurvedic approach to the care for your particular body type; or use them as a quick check before working with the lengthier questionaires.

VATA

_____ thin, light-bone build
_____ dry hair, skin, and nails
_____ thinks, speaks, moves quickly
_____ enthusiastic, imaginative, sensitive, not very practical
_____ catches on quickly, forgets easily
_____ prone to worry and mood swings
_____ hates the cold, loves the sun
_____ tires easily
_____ hungry anytime
_____ nothing in life is routine; loves to travel and change
_____ loves crunchy, salty snacks
_____ spends money easily

PITTA

_____ medium, athletic build—blonde, red or prematurely grey hair; fair or freckled in complexion
_____ penetrating eyes, direct in speech
_____ confident, courageous, aggressive
_____ intelligent, insightful, ambitious

_____ leader, organizer, idealistic, brainstormer
_____ great planner, self-disciplined
_____ tendency to anger easily and be overly critical
_____ tired by excessive heat
_____ enjoys physical and mental challenges
_____ hates to miss a meal, especially lunch; eats volumes
_____ loves spicy, oily food, or ice cream
_____ spends on luxuries

KAPHA
_____ square, powerful build
_____ exotic, heavy features, lustrous hair
_____ graceful, relaxed
_____ tolerant, compassionate, loyal, calm
_____ excellent memory
_____ can be dull, boring, and greedy or overly possessive
_____ likes to sleep a lot
_____ hates uncomfortable surroundings
_____ reliable worker
_____ enjoys gourmet foods and all types of comforts
_____ likes their own nest
_____ loves sweet, sticky, creamy treats
_____ makes and sows money well

Single Dosha Dominant

In the above section *On Identifying Attributes,* if one of the categories (Vata, Pitta, Kapha) has twice as many checkmarks as the other two categories, chances are you're a single dosha type. This is considered very unusual so you may want to check through the charts again when personal circumstances or seasons change.

Dual Dosha Dominant

Most people are in this category. Here you can identify strongly and fairly evenly with the attributes of two doshas and the third to a far lesser extent. Notice how one or the other of the doshas may become dominant or imbalanced with the change of season or personal situation.

Tridosha Type

This is rare. If you identify equally with each dosha type, you may be correct. Check physical attributes again carefully. You might like to ask for a second opinion. Select treatments for skin, hair, and nails symptomatically; e.g., if skin is cool, dry and rough, treat for Vata. If hair is red, straight, and oily, treat for Pitta. If nails are strong, square, and thick, treat for Kapha.

No matter which dosha is dominant, (single, dual or tridosha) all have wonderful qualities as well as inherent difficulties. Which type is in fashion has changed with the times and with varying cultural views. Whether or not you are a match with what is currently considered attractive will be over-shadowed by the real strength of beauty that will become available to you through Ayurvedic care. Appropriate care of your prakruti will bring grace to your body, light to your eyes, luster to your skin, and joy to your heart.

Choosing Treatments for Mixed Dosha Types
- If you are slightly more Vata than Pitta . . .
  Treat for Pitta when the skin is oilier, warmer, or inflamed.
  Treat for Vata when the skin is drier, colder, and more sallow.

- If you are slightly more Vata than Kapha . . .
  Treat for Kapha when the skin is oilier, whiter, or more puffy.
  Treat for Vata when the skin is drier or more sallow.

- If you are slightly more Pitta than Vata . . .
  Treat for Vata when the skin is drier, cooler, or more rough, and

the hair is drier and coarser.

Treat for Pitta when the skin is oilier, warmer, moister, or inflamed.

• If you are slightly more Pitta than Kapha . . .

Treat for Kapha when the skin is oilier, cooler, whiter, and less moist.

Treat for Pitta when skin is warmer, more moist, sensitive, and inflamed.

• If you are slightly more Kapha than Vata . . .

Treat for Vata when the skin is drier or more sallow.

Treat for Kapha when the skin is oilier, more congested, or whiter looking.

• If you are slightly more Kapha than Pitta . . .

Treat for Pitta when the skin is less oily, moister, warmer, or inflamed.

Treat for Kapha when skin is oilier, cooler, whiter, less moist.

As well as your prakruti or constitution, you also have your condition or vikruti to consider. This is the more changeable aspect of your being and is most influenced by external circumstances; climate and diet being the strongest influences. So, pay attention to your climate as a key for treatment choices, too.

Hot, sunny weather will naturally increase Pitta and decrease Vata and Kapha

Cold, dry, windy or little changeable weather will increase Vata and decrease Pitta and Kapha (if not excessively cold, i.e. Kapha)

Cold, humid, foggy, cloudy, rainy, snowy weather will increase Kapha, decrease Pitta and Vata (if not too cold, i.e. Vata)

THE ROLE OF THE DHATUS
IN PHYSICAL BEAUTY

There are seven *dhatus* or body tissues that give shape and form to the body. These seven are *rasa* (tissue fluids), *rakta* (red blood cells), *mamsa* (skeletal muscle), *meda* (fat and connective tissue), *asthi* (bones), *majja* (bone marrow), and *shukra* (reproductive tissue). Their nature is to nourish and support one another, rasa nourishing rakta, rakta nourishing mamsa, and so on. Therefore, if a problem exists in one of the seven dhatus, those down the line also start to suffer, as they are also not being properly supported.

Each of the dhatus also nourish and support a subsidiary tissue or *upadhatu* and produce waste products or *malas*. The upadhatus neither nourish each other nor any other tissue for that matter. The relationships between dhatus, upadhatus, and malas are as follows. What will also be included here are the ways the dhatus influence our overall physiological being.

• Rasa supports colostrum and menstrual blood and produces mucous as waste. As it receives nutrients from the digestive process, Rasa helps to nourish the entire body.

• Rakta supports the blood vessels and tendons and produces bile as waste. It also brings oxygen to the tissues and takes carbon dioxide away, invigorating the entire body.

• Mamsa supports subcutaneous fat and the skin and produces wastes emitted from the body's orifices. As mamsa is associated with skeletal muscles, it is responsible for giving the body its smooth contours.

• Meda supports fat and flat muscle, producing sweat as waste. Being slippery in nature, meda is responsible for lubrication within the body.

• Asthi supports teeth and produces body hair, beard and nails as waste.

21

TABLE 1

DHATU	UPADHATU	MALAS	PHYSICAL FUNCTION	POSITIVE EMOTIONAL EXPRESSION
RASA (chyle, lymph, blood plasma)	Stanya (mammary glands) Artava (mentrual blood & lactation)	mucous	nourishment	satisfaction with food, compassion, exaltation, lust-for-life
RAKTA (red blood cells)	Sira (blood vessels) Kardrara (muscle tendons)	bile	invigoration	enthusiasm, vitality, excitement
MAMSA (skeletal muscle)	Snayu (flat muscles) Twacha (skin)	wastes that accumulate in orifices; ear wax, navel lint, nasal mucous, smegma	covering the skeleton	courageous, protected, forgiving, well coordinated
MEDA (fat in limbs and torso)	Snaya (subcutaneous fat)	sweat	lubrication	able to commit in love or friendship
ASTHI (bones)	Danta (teeth)	nails, body, hair & beard	support	supported, grounded, strong, purposeful
MAJJA (bone marrow)	(head hair)	lachrymal secretion	"filling" space	firm in sense of self, able to protect self with clear, calm eyes
SHUKRA (male & female reproductive fluids)	Ojas (produces aura & controls immunity)	(none)	reproduction	wish for children or strong creativity, able to make mark in the world

TABLE 1 (Cont.)

EMOTIONAL EXPRESSION WHEN UNBALANCED	RELATED BEAUTY CONDITIONS WHEN UNBALANCED	FOODS THAT AGGRAVATE	FOODS THAT BENEFIT	SPECIAL TREATMENTS TO BALANCE
suspicion, cheated, frustrated, abused; lack of faith, of taste, lack of self-confidence	fatigue, depression, overall dryness, anemia, heavy feeling, clogged veins, premature aging, emmaciation, PMS, aches & pain	fatty, sugary foods	sea vegetables (esp. agar agar), fruit & veg. juices, aloe vera	fasting
anger, irritability, violence, lack of love	dryness, dull skin, varicose veins, rashes, acne, bruising	acid producing foods	minerals (esp. iron-rich foods	fasting, laxatives, blood-letting, deep breathing
defenseless, unsupported, unforgiving, poorly organized	weakness & immaciation in muscles, eczema, dermatitis, cysts, psoriasis, abscesses	low protein diets	quality protein, all essential amino acids	surgery, cauterization
clinging, emotionally ready	dry skin, obesity or immaciation, dry or oily hair & nails, heavy breasts, smelly sweat	heavy, fatty foods	essential fatty acids	fasting, exercise, sweating, vomiting
ungrounded, weak, low energy	osteoporosis, poor posture, cavities in teeth, hair loss, beard on women	excess protein, refined sugars	mineral rich food, sesame seeds, sea vegetables	pancha karma, esp. basti
emptiness of mind, feeling worthless, lifeless eyes, persuasive but weak, aggrandizing	sunken or protruding eyes, heaving, sticky eyes, numbness	stress when eating	Vit. B-rich foods, proteins, lecithin	elimination of excess doshas
weak creativity, vulnerability	difficulties with libido	pre-occupation with fears & anxieties while eating	milk, ghee, rejuvenative herbs (i.e. shatavari, ashwagandha)	exercise, sweet & bitter foods, sex

It creates the supportive structure for the musculature.

• Majja supports head hair and helps produce mother's milk as its waste or by-product. Majja is what helps to fill in the spaces of the body.

• Shukra supports ojas, the glow of health and produces no wastes. It is responsible for reproduction.

Looking on Table 1 (pps. 22-23), will help you to make these connections more easily.

To understand the connection between the dhatus and upadhatus and wastes, let us take an example: skin.

Skin is called the cream of rasa, but actually rasa, rakta, and mamsa dhatus have to be in good condition to produce beautiful skin. Good digestion and correct selection of foods determine the health of rasa dhatu. Mineral-rich foods and a good supply of oxygen and lack of toxins in the blood determine the health of rakta dhatu. Clean, well nourished blood and regular exercise supports the health of mamsa dhatu. Thus, diet, digestion, air, and exercise can be seen to be important in the condition of the skin. This is how a knowledge of dhatus helps us understand how to bring beauty to a particular tissue. If this does not happen, examining the upadhatus and malas can prove useful in finding which of the dhatus needs attention. Let's take another example: nails.

The condition of asthi dhatu determines the condition of the nails in that mineral rich food that nourishes bone tissue also produces gleaming teeth and strong nails. Yet, as asthi dhatu is supported by other dhatus, problems in the nails can reflect problems in rasa, rakta, mamsa or meda dhatus—those that support asthi. This explains how nails can be examined to determine the internal state of the body. For example, vertical ridges on the nails show malabsorption, a problem in rasa dhatu. (Check the nail care section, p. 144, for more details on the conditions and treatments for nails.)

As regards other aspects of physical beauty, strong majja dhatu produces strong, glossy hair—a commonly accepted sign of good health. And, the product of shukra dhatu that is the glow of vitality, ojas, is dependent on the health of all the tissues in the body which is why we can say that internal health is essential for radiant beauty.

Table 1 (pps. 22-23) will help you to keep correlations correctly in mind. Included in this are the emotional states associated with each of the dhatus. For the condition of the dhatus not only influences the overall condition of the body, but also the state of mind. Health and balance in the dhatus produces pleasant, attractive ways of being. At the same time, the power of mind balancing and enhancing activities such as prayer, meditation, and acting in ways that evoke feelings of love, compassion, and peacefulness will, in turn, help to balance the dhatus. Of course, the optimal way of living ones life is to cultivate positive physical and mental states. In that way, you can't go wrong, the results of which will radiate from your appearance and demeanor.

The Importance of Malas

Ayurveda strongly stresses that elimination of wastes is as important to the health and beauty of the body as the nourishment it receives. Keeping the tissues cleansed of wastes and facilitating their regular elimination through normal channels is the key to freshness and vitality. Only a clean body can be at its peak and utilize the nutrients it receives, likewise, only an open mind is free to enjoy the world.

There are various means to help support the health of the dhatus that one will find throughout this volume. At the same time, one of the best ways to accomplish this is by strengthening *Ojas*.

The Nature of Ojas

Ojas is the fine essence of all the dhatus and the superfine essence of *shukra dhatu*. It manifests in our physical being as the sap of life energy, giving power to the heart muscle, regulating the heart's own natural pacemaker, providing nourishment to all the muscles, maintaining the action of the liver and kidneys, and providing us with a strong immune system. On a subtle level, it is the life force that can be felt when touching a vital individual and sensing the fresh brightness they project. When ojas is strong the body is strong, firm, and flexible; the skin is smooth, clear, and lustrous; the hair is thick, manageable, and shiny; the face looks calm with a natural smile; the body posture is relaxed and movement is naturally graceful; and the voice is melodious and speech is kind. The *soma,* or substance ojas produces in the brain, is the source for the capacity to love. It is the subtle, physical manifestation of what allows the mind to express itself with natural compassion, loving kindness, peacefulness, and creativity—the highest attributes of beauty. With spiritual practice, ojas is transformed to strengthen the aura, thus giving the adept's body a deep radiance. Spiritual practices such as meditation, prayer, and chanting are also considered very strengthening to ojas. Consider how many religious paintings portray the glowing quality of the forms and faces of gods, saints, and holy people. This glow is ojas.

When ojas is lost or destroyed, the opposite of health becomes apparent. All the qualities we associate with a lack of vitality, both physical and mental, manifest. Here are some of the factors that can contribute to the destruction of ojas:

• pursuing a lifestyle that aggravates vata dosha
• eating de-vitalized foods; overly processed, microwaved, old, stale, junk food, etc.
• air flight, high speed cars, fast, intense sports with no relaxation to balance
• computers, T.V. and low level radiation
• loud music
• constant distraction
• over exercising
• fasting too long or too often
• being caught up in conflicting emotions: fear, worry, anger, sorrow, grasping, impatience

- overwork
- lack of faith or confidence
- excessive sex
- unnatural environments
- illness

Although ojas can be destroyed, it can also be regained and strengthened. Aside from religious and spiritual practices, there are natural, everyday ways to increase ojas. Following a lifestyle suitable to keep your body in balance is central; simple attention to appropriate loving care. Then there are specific remedies. Warm, raw milk and ghee (clarified butter) are highly valued as foods because they directly nourish ojas as do rejuvenative herbs such as *shatavari, ashwaganda,* and *guduchi.* (One cup of raw milk, one teaspoon of ghee, and one-half teaspoon of herbs makes a wonderful nightcap.) A quiet holiday with country walks, good food, rest, and sound sleep can do wonders. From an Ayurvedic point of view, it is the regeneration of ojas in the body that makes a person coming from such a holiday look rested, refreshed, calm, and radiant. It becomes apparent that many aspects of modern life are destructive to ojas. Therefore diet, lifestyle, and spiritual practice are essential elements in the restoration of ojas, our vitality and natural beauty.

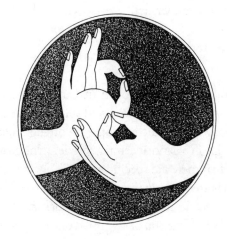

DAILY ROUTINES TO ENHANCE BEAUTY

"As is a man's will, so is his action.
As is his action, so he becomes."
Brihadaranyaka U 4.5

The following section contains detailed information about how to manage many aspects of daily life to create harmony in the body. Such information should be treated as guidelines for living, to be adopted gradually as circumstances allow. The intention is not to be restrictive, but to appeal to the basic nature of the body that, when given appropriate options and time to adjust, prefers routine over chaos and desires space and freedom to develop a truly creative way of being. Please remember that too much change at once—even in a positive direction—is hard for the body to handle. Change a few things at a time. Reflect on the results. If they seem to make a sufficient difference in how you look and feel, chances are these new ways will become a part of your daily life. This is how real discipline arises; a discipline that arises from true self will add a sense of joy in doing what works. Using Ayurvedic principles as tools for self-exploration in this way, you can become your own healer and truly be in command of your own potential.

The Importance of Diet for Beauty

"As long as we are not living in harmony
with nature and our constitution, we
cannot expect ourselves to be really healed.
Ayurveda gives us the means."
—David Frawley

29

According to Ayurveda, it is the perfect digestion and assimilation of our food together with the regular and efficient evacuation of wastes that is essential for beauty. These form the cornerstone for a strong, well-balanced, and beautiful being. Together they are responsible for producing clear skin, bright eyes, glossy hair, strong nails, stamina, clarity, and a gentle, compassionate nature. Any food, no matter how perfect, that is improperly digested forms toxic wastes called *"ama."* Ama, in turn, clogs the system, impeding good digestion—compounding the problem by creating blockages in vital channels and clouding the mind.

Good digestion is enhanced by intelligent selection and skillful preparation of foods, plus a mindful attitude when eating. Before talking specifically about food preparation and selection, we shall first look at general guidelines for helping digestion.

General Guidelines for Helping Digestion

• When there are any signs of improperly digested food or ama, such as bad breath, heavily coated tongue, gas, cloudy urine, nausea, or digestive upset, it is best to give the system time to clean and balance itself by fasting for a day or at least skipping a meal until a sense of appetite returns.

• Never eat when angry, depressed, bored, upset, or exhausted.

• Bathe before eating. If this is not practical, wash your hands and face.

• Eat at home as much as possible. Food prepared with love and pure intention to benefit others is always better energy than food produced in a restaurant which is intended to turn a profit. Traditionally, cooks in India were chosen from the priestly class to ensure that good energy went into the food.

• Eat alone or with friends and family in whose company you can completely relax.

• Eat in a quiet, clean place. Facing east when eating maximizes the energy for digestion.

• Listen to classical music or Indian music designed to aid digestion. Both are helpful in setting the mood for dining.

• Sip warm water with your meal to aid digestion. Never drink ice water or milk with your meal.

• Use ginger to help spur the appetite. Prepare it by chopping it finely and mixing with a little lemon juice and a small amount of rock salt. Pitta types usually don't need this and so long as their appetite is strong, they are better off without it.

• Minimize raw foods. Cooked foods are generally easier to digest.

• Give thanks for what you are about to eat and extend that good feeling into your food so that it serves each cell of your being.

• Quiet while eating is best, except for pleasant background music. It is said that the quality of conversation after the meal reflects the nature and quality of the meal, whereas conversation during the meal is a distraction to good digestion.

• Eat only as much as would fit into your two hands cupped together.

• Eat foods of all six tastes: sweet, sour, salty, bitter, pungent, astringent—varying portions to suit your doshic balance.

• Eat fresh, local, seasonal foods whenever possible.

• Avoid excessive sour or fermented foods, especially yeasted bread.

• Give thanks at the end of the meal.

• Clean the mouth, rinse the eyes, and take a short walk.

• Leave 3 to 6 hours between meals.

• Try to keep regular meal times.

• Avoid sex, deep study, or sleep for at least two hours after eating, especially in the evening. Watching T.V. during or directly after meals will inhibit proper digestion.

Guidelines for Food Selection

When the *rishis* wrote about diet, they were living in a simpler, less polluted world. Times have changed and many issues need consideration when addressing diet. The suggestions that follow are not necessarily traditional, but are in keeping with the spirit of Ayurveda.

• Select organic foods when possible. Not only do you avoid potentially poisonous chemicals that block and age tissues, but also organic foods are richer in nutrients, especially trace minerals—important to skin, hair, nails, and temperament.

• Eat foods that grow in the area in which you live or within a 400-mile radius so they can be from a similar climate zone. Foods that grow well in your area will help you to keep well and look good. As they flourish in your local area, so will you.

• Eat foods that are in season so they are freshest and naturally most suited to the climate in the particular time that you are in. For example, greens in spring, zucchini in summer, carrots in fall, acorn squash in winter. Fresh foods are fullest in vitality and give you more energy.

• Pay attention to selecting foods appropriate to your dosha. Also, take note of the season and time of day when a particular dosha is naturally higher and adjust your selection accordingly. Pay particular attention to food selection when you travel or eat out.

Vata is higher in the autumn and winter, and daily, in the afternoon.

Pitta is higher in summer and daily, at midday.

Kapha is higher in the spring and daily, in the early morning and evening.

More information regarding dosha dominance and food selection follows:

• Eat freshly prepared foods as much as possible. Fresh leftovers (no more than one day old) are preferable to fast foods, however.

• Avoid poor food combinations, such as . . .

　　very hot and very cold foods
　　raw and cooked foods
　　milk and fish
　　milk and meat

• Avoid microwaves. This form of cooking disperses rather than condenses energy and is thus weakening over time. This has been scientifically and empirically proven.

• Food should look and smell appetizing. Pleasant garnishes and an attractive table setting also help to instill a sense of harmony at the table.

• Drink spring water or purified water. Avoid distilled water as it is devoid of all minerals and can leach them from your system, weakening bones, teeth, hair, nails, and skin. However, there are currently available mineral formulations that can be added to distilled water to rectify this problem.

• Chew each mouthful of food well—at least until it is liquidy.

• Finish the meal with lassi, a drink made with yoghurt that should have live acidophilus bacteria, helpful to digestion. Modern diets are harsh on intestinal flora and often cause imbalances that lead to digestive problems. Acidophilus helps to restore the balance. Homemade yoghurt is best. Use recipes described in the section on your dosha to best suit your needs.

Eating According to Your Dosha

The attention given to treating people as individuals is one of the greatest gifts of the Ayurvedic approach to health and beauty. This is particularly evident in the selection of one's optimum diet.

Rather than approaching diet from the standpoint of calories or particular nutrients in foods as is done in the west, an Ayurvedic diet is based more on the intuitive sense of what is attractive to the individual by color, smell, temperature, taste, and texture; trusting that when the body is in balance, it will be attracted to foods by its own innate intelligence. This works well when we are healthy. However, because there are so many influences in our modern world which throw us off balance, it is useful to have some more defined guidelines.

Foods in Ayurveda are classified by their qualities or "gunas" and taste or "rasa." There are six main gunas . . .

heavy	light
dry	oily
hot	cold

and there are six rasas . . .

sweet	bitter
sour	pungent or spicy
salty	astringent or "puckering"

The qualities and taste of the food that are best for a particular dosha will be those which help to counteract the qualities of the dosha. That is, foods for a particular dosha are there not to enhance or make the dosha more that way, but to balance its tendencies with opposite qualities and resultant tendencies. For example: Vata is dry cold, and irregular by nature, so foods that balance Vata are moist, warming, and taken at regular mealtimes.

This being said, however, all tastes and qualities should be present in one meal, the portions of each varying to balance the dominant dosha of the individual. This makes for the most satisfying dining experience and curbs cravings for over-eating and snacking. Such balancing may seem complicated, but it is no more cumbersome than the experience many people have of eating a meal and then feeling that something is missing or such-and-such would just round off the meal. Paying attention to the gunas and taste in your meal helps you to easily plan the perfect meal ahead of time. Use your imagination, intuition, and intelligence when planning a meal. Cooking is an art and takes time and patience to perfect.

Many types of diet have been proposed as being "perfect"—the answer to all of our ills. Ayurveda teaches us differently. One person's meat may be another person's poison. What is wonderfully healthy for Vata people is not always helpful to Kapha people. For example, Vata people do well with a healthy bowl of hot grain cereal and hot milk for breakfast. It grounds and gives them energy for the entire morning. If a Kapha person were to eat the same, he or she would feel heavy and probably fall asleep on the way to work.

This being said, although there is variation of diet among the various dosha dominances, Ayurveda honors what has basically worked as the most life-sustaining foods and food proportions for humans over the course of history; a diet of 40-60% whole cereal grains, 30-50% fresh fruits and vegetables, and 10-20% high quality proteins, with specific types of each food and proportions being in accordance with dosha dominance. This approach also serves to simplify your meal plan!

Before looking at specific dietary recommendations for the various doshas, there are times of day that will naturally increase certain doshas in the body. Knowing this helps you to plan the best times for meals to keep your dosha in balance.

6:00AM—10:00AM KAPHA TIME—Take breakfast before 8:00AM. Breakfast should be light. Vata people need a nourishing breakfast. Kapha people can skip it altogether or have a beverage. Pitta people can do with a light breakfast so they are not ravenous by lunchtime.

10:00AM—2:00PM PITTA TIME—Best hours for lunch or brunch. Pitta people do best with an early lunch. For them, lunch should be the most substantial meal if possible. Small meal for Vatas with snacks mid-morning and afternoon and Kaphas should have a light main meal.

2:00PM—6:00PM VATA TIME—Vata and Pitta people may like a snack at 3:00PM—4:00PM to sustain their energy. All doshas should try to have their evening meal before 6:00PM if possible. Dinner should be lighter than lunch, if possible.

6:00PM—10:00PM KAPHA TIME—The body's digestive ability slows towards evening. Vata people may need an evening snack. Pitta people can eat a little fruit if they stay up late. Kapha people should not have anything except a cup of hot tea. One should refrain from eating for at least two hours before sleep.

If you are predominantly one dosha, then follow the guidelines for that dosha. If you have mixed-dosha dominance, then vary your diet according to your needs and the season.

Remember: These are only dietary suggestions. Try them, work with them, reflect on them and find your own balance. Be flexible and always try to enjoy what you eat.

Vata-Pitta types—follow a vata diet for fall and winter and a Pitta diet for spring and summer. Go easy on spices.

Pitta-Kapha types—follow a Pitta diet in late spring to fall and Kapha diet from late fall through the spring. Go easy on cold foods.

Vata-Kapha types—follow a Vata diet for summer and fall and Kapha diet for winter and spring.

DIET FOR VATA

General Considerations

• As people with dominant Vata dosha have both unpredictable appetites and an inherent loathing of routine, eating quality food in sufficient quantity by eating more frequently is useful, as long as there is hunger.

• Key qualities of Vata diet are warm, heavy, moistening, nourishing, nurturing, soothing, satisfying, and grounding. Warm foods are best, especially stews and simple one-dish meals. Avoid a great variety at one meal.

• Use mild spices and a little salt to help prime digestion.

• Eating at home is best. Eating fast food is the very worst choice.

• Be aware of allergies. Vata people do not tolerate nightshades (potatoes, tomatoes, peppers, eggplant) and are often lactose intolerant.

• Avoid eating when nervous, anxious, afraid, deep in thought, or worried or otherwise distracted.

• As Vata digestion is the least strong, pay attention to eating when eating; avoid watching T.V., listening to radio, reading, etc.

• Eat with people who take pleasure in eating in a calm, tidy, clean, and spacious feeling atmosphere.

• Skipping meals is not good, but overeating is worse. Avoid "pigging out" on anything. Excess is never good for Vata types.

• Vata is increased by age, autumn season, afternoon time, travel, loud noise, cold and wind. Be particularly careful with diet at these times or when in these situations.

• Qualities of food that balance Vata are: sweet, heavy, sour, salty, oily, warm. Take proportionately more of these.

• Qualities of food that unbalance Vata are: pungent, bitter, astringent, light, dry, cold. Take less of these and less frequently.

Daily Eating Routine for Vata Types

• Eat 3 or 4 small meals a day at regular times. Leave at least 2 hours between small meals or snacks.
• Eat a good breakfast. Take a hot milky drink at night to help with sound sleep.
• Daily, take 5-6 servings of some whole grain or whole grain product, plus . . .
    1-2 servings of high quality protein
    2-3 servings of fresh cooked vegetables
    1 serving of fruit
    drink plenty of liquid
• Vata dominance is responsible for an irregular digestive power. Watch out for signs of poor digestion, like gas, bloating, heaviness in the head and limbs, restlessness, lethargy, or poor elimination (constipation). If such symptoms arise, eat very lightly until the digestion is strengthened.

Shopping List for Vata
(reduce and photocopy, take a copy with you when you shop and put one copy on the refrigerator):
* means occasionally.

GRAINS: brown rice, sweet brown rice, basmati rice, wild rice, oats (cooked), *amaranth, whole wheat cereals and pastas, udon noodles

LEGUMES: split mung, red lentils, aduki, tofu, soy beverage

ANIMAL PRODUCTS: eggs, chicken, turkey, fresh- and salt-water fish, shrimp

VEGETABLES: (in season is best) asparagus, acorn squash, artichokes, beets, butternut squash, carrots, cucumber, green beans, hot peppers, leeks, mustard greens, okra, olives, onions, parsnips, pumpkins, radish, rutabaga, summer squashes, sweet potato

DAIRY: unhomogenized cows milk, *goat milk, cottage cheese, buttermilk, soft cheese, hard cheese, yoghurt, *ice cream, *sour cream

FRUITS: apricots, avocados, bananas (ripe), berries (sweet), cherries, coconut, dates, fresh figs, grapefruit, kiwi, lemon, limes, *mangoes, melons, oranges, papayas, peaches, pineapple, plum, rhubarb, raisins (soaked)

NUTS and SEEDS: almonds, *brazils, *cashews, *hazelnuts, *pecans, *pine nuts, *pistachio, pumpkin, sesame, sunflower, *walnuts

SWEETENERS: barley malt, brown rice syrup, *ghur, *jaggery, fruit juice concentrates, honey, maple syrup, molasses, *sucanat, *sugar cane juice

CONDIMENTS and PICKLES: lemon juice, lime juice, gomasio (sesame seed and sea salt mixture), japanese ginger pickle, mayonnaise, miso, natural soy sauce, sweet pickles, sweet chutney, sea vegetables, sesame seeds, and umeboshi plums

OILS and SPICES: asafoetida, ajwan, garlic, ginger, mustard oil, sesame oil (All spices are good if used moderately and cooked properly. Refer to *The Ayurvedic Cookbook*, by Amadea Morningstar.)

DRINKS: Aloe Vera juice, fruit and vegetable juices, smoothies, coffee substitutes (Cafix, Roma, Pero), herbals teas (chamomile, lavender, licorice, fennel, ginger, raspberry), vegetable broths

When Eating Out . . .

- Avoid strong liquors and beer.
- Warmed medicinal wine or diluted table wine is O.K.
- Eat soup instead of salad or use a creamy or oily dressing to make the salad more digestible and less rough for the system.
- Sip hot water with the meal, avoiding ice water.
- Go for a warm dessert or hot tea at the end of the meal.
- If you *must* have ice cream, drink hot tea with clove and cardamon later.

Preparation Tips for Vata Diet

GRAINS: Most grains are useful, as they are warming and grounding. Some are too drying for regular use. Yeasted breads and pastries are best avoided as they cause gas and disturb the digestive system.

Use a variety of whole grains to avoid developing allergies. Cook grains with a little more water than the regular 1 cup grain to 2 cups water ratio, adding a little salt, clarified butter or oil, slices of ginger, and a pinch of ghur (Indian raw sugar).

LEGUMES: Beans are an excellent source of protein, but can be a challenge to digest. Processing by splitting the beans and removing the hull makes them easier to digest which is why split mung and red lentils are so popular in Indian cuisine. If beans cause gas formation, they are increasing Vata dosha. This problem can be helped by:
• soaking whole beans overnight and changing the water before cooking (adding kombu seaweed for overnight cooking will also help).
• cooking for long periods of time with the lid off so Vata causing products can 'bubble' off. All day, on an open fire, (Navajo-style) is best. A crockpot for beans is better than a pressure cooker in the modern kitchen.
• use turmeric, cumin, coriander, ginger, garlic, and asafoetida as standard spices when cooking beans.
• eat beans in small quantities (10-20% of meal, proportionately), chewing very well.

VEGETABLES: Cooking vegetables is the best way to improve their digestibility for Vata people; stir fry, stew, or bake and serve with sauce. Raw vegetables and salads can be made more digestible by quick pickling, pressed with a little salt, or serving them with an oily or creamy dressing.

MEATS: As beans are difficult for Vata people to digest and dairy products often cause allergenic reactions, meat and eggs, correctly prepared, provide a vital source of protein.

Meats are best prepared with ginger, garlic, turmeric, and black pepper, cooked thoroughly and served in stews or with sauce or gravy. White meats, fresh fish, or wild game are best. Lamb or beef is used if real grounding is needed.

DAIRY: If well tolerated, milk and milk products are a strengthening, body-building food. Milk, itself, is most easily digested by Vata people when it is heated and mixed with spice. Other examples are . . .
• Lassi—yoghurt mixed 1:3 with water and a little lemon juice, pinch of salt, slice of fresh ginger, powdered cumin and coriander—taken after meals
• hot milk toddy with ghee, ginger, and a little honey
• cheese fondue
• spicy cheese sauce with chili

FRUIT: Fruits that are sweet, moist, and well ripened are suitable. Dried fruit is too dry unless soaked and cooked in a compote, preferably with ginger and cinnamon. Cooked fruit is best eaten as dessert approximately twenty minutes after the rest of the meal. Raw fruits can disturb digestion unless they are eaten alone as a snack or before a meal as a light appetizer or chutney. This applies especially to fruits in the melon family.

NUTS and SEEDS: Nuts are best soaked and cooked into dishes or blended into nut butters for the Vata digestive system. Smoothies with nut milk are a great snack for Vatas on the go. Also, 10 almonds that have been soaked and skinned provide all the nutrients a body needs for one day—a popular Ayurvedic snack.

SWEETENERS: Honey in moderation and never cooked into things is best; just add to foods for sweetness. Vatas most easily suffer from fluctuating blood sugar levels, thus should totally avoid white sugar.

CONDIMENTS and PICKLES: Pickles, if they are more salty than sour, can perk up a Vata appetite and aid in digestion.

Condiments help provide variety, excitement and interest to the simple meals that are best for Vatas, but are a little against their tendencies to want excessive stimulation. Sea vegetables are particularly useful as they are very high in minerals which help build rich skin, hair, and strong nails—often what Vatas need.

SPICE: Most spices are good unless in excess or extremely strong in taste. Too much hot spice can dry Vata people too much or cause sweat that dispels body heat.

DRINKS: Drinks are best warm or at room temperature. Coffee and tea are too stimulating, as is alcohol. Fizzy drinks can be too gassy. Fruit and vegetable juices are O.K. but in excess are too sweet and do not provide enough fiber for good digestion. They are good alternatives to total fasting if there is a lot of toxic build-up. Herbal teas made of the herbs and spices that benefit Vatas are good to warm the body, help digestion, and calm the nerves.

DIET for PITTA

General Considerations

• People with a dominant Pitta dosha usually have a strong appetite that needs to be satisfied regularly. Unsatisfied appetite leads to intense hunger and to outbursts of irritation, even anger.

• Key qualities for Pitta diet are cool, slightly dry (not soggy or oily) and a little heavy. Avoid salt.

• Eat main meals or at least a good size meal at midday.

• Avoid late night eating. Fresh fruit or vegetables are the best evening snack if appetite demands.

• Eating with an attitude of calm and gratitude is particularly helpful.

• Avoid eating when angry, irritated, or in competitive situations. Business lunches might be a bad idea.

• Pitta's strong digestion can lead to the development of abusive habits that cause problems eventually, i.e. over-eating, eating excessively greasy foods, or excessively rich or hot, spicy food.

• Avoid salty, greasy, overly cooked, excessively rich, heavily spiced, or sour foods as well as caffeine, red meat, many eggs, alcohol, and sugar.

• Pitta is increased by summer, at midday and midnight, intense heat, excessive sunlight. Be most mindful at these times.

• Qualities of food that balance Pitta: sweet, astringent, bitter, cool, heavy, dry. Take proportionately more of these.

• Qualities of food that unbalance Pitta: pungent, hot, sour, light, salty, oily. Take less of these and less frequently.

Daily Eating Routine for Pitta Types

• Eat 3 meals a day at regular times, leaving at least a 4-hour gap between meals.

• Eat a light breakfast and take an early lunch.

• Take 4-5 servings of whole grains
    1½-2 servings of high quality protein
    3-4 servings for fresh vegetables
    1-1½ servings fresh fruit or more
    Drink liquid moderately (more after exercise).

Shopping List for Pitta
*(reduce and/or copy and take with you when you shop
and place one on the refrigerator)*
* means occasionally

GRAINS: barley, white basmati rice, wheat, whole wheat tortillas, wheat pastas, rice cakes

LEGUMES: Any beans except red lentil, tempeh

ANIMAL PRODUCTS: chicken (white meat), turkey (white meat), egg whites, *fresh water fish

VEGETABLES: acorn squash, artichoke, asparagus, bell pepper, broccoli, brussels sprouts, burdock, butternut squash, *black olives, cabbage, cilantro, corn, cauliflower, collards, celery, cucumber, green beans, jicama, kale, lettuce, mushroom, okra, peas, parsley, parsnips, potato, rutabaga, sweet potato, summer squash, *watercress, zucchini

DAIRY: unsalted butter, cottage cheese, soft cheese, cow and goat milk, ghee, *ice cream, *yoghurt

FRUITS: apples, apricots. avocado, berries (sweet), coconut, dates, figs, grapes, mango, melons, oranges, pears, pineapple, plum, pomegranate, prune, raisin, watermelon

NUTS and SEEDS: coconut, pumpkin, sunflower

DRINKS: aloe vera juice, fruit or vegetable juice, coconut milk, milk smoothies, Cafix, Roma, Pero, vegetable broth,and herbal teas such as barley, chamomile, fennel, hibiscus, jasmine, lavender, mint, raspberry, rose petal

SWEETENERS: barley malt syrup, brown rice syrup, maple syrup, juice concentrates, fructose, sugar cane juice, *sucanat

CONDIMENTS: *sea vegetables, lemon, lime, lime pickle, mango chutney, mango pickle, soy mayonnaise, soy sauce, *yoghurt

OILS: avocado, coconut, olive, sunflower, soy, walnut, *sesame

SPICES: coriander, cumin, dill, fennel, mint, neem, peppermint, rosewater, saffron, turmeric

Preparation Tips for Pitta Diet

GRAINS: Grains are balancing to Pitta dosha as they are filling, satisfying, but not too heavy. Barley and basmati rice are best.

LEGUMES: Pitta people seem, in practice, to need the greatest amount of protein to fuel their high drive lifestyle. All beans are good, with the exception of tempeh, red and black lentils. Prepare as described in Vata preparation tips.

ANIMAL FOOD: Although Pitta types need a good amount of protein, they are best suited to a totally vegetarian diet. Most meats are either too fatty or heat producing. Small amounts of poultry and fresh water fish are alright. Heavier meat consumption can make the Pitta personality too intense and make them attracted to alcohol and drugs for recreation and relaxation.

DAIRY: If well tolerated, milk products, with the exception of hard or aged cheeses, help nourish and cool Pitta people. Sour or very salty dairy products should be avoided. Yoghurt may be taken as lassi after a meal (Recipe: 1 part yoghurt to 3 part warm water, maple syrup or ghur [Indian Sugar], cilantro [also called Chinese or Italian parsley], cardamon)

VEGETABLES: Quantities of vegetables are good for Pitta types. Their high metabolism uses vitamins and minerals quickly, especially Vitamin A. A salad including bitter greens like endive, arugula, and parsley can help curb over-eating. Tomatoes, radishes, and garlic are best totally avoided.

FRUITS: Sweet fruits are good, especially fresh figs and grapes (figs are not recommended when pregnant, however). A little lemon and lime for zest is fine. Fruits make the best evening snack.

NUTS and SEEDS: Generally they are too hot and oily, with the exception of coconut milk which is delightful in cooking. Sunflower seeds are fine and occasionally pumpkin seeds.

SWEETENERS: Pitta types tolerate sugar sweet taste the best. This is another thing they need to be cautious about eating in quantity over the long term. Honey and molasses should be avoided. These sweeteners can even be the cause of rashes for the Pitta person in summer.

SPICES: Use those on the shopping list. As you become familiar with Ayurvedic principles, you will be able to widen your selection. For example, black pepper can be balanced by using it with cilantro.

DRINKS: An occasional beer is better than wine. Hard liquor should be avoided (So should salted nuts and pretzels, often served at bars, as it leads to more drinking.)

A little black tea can be tolerated, but coffee is best avoided entirely.

When Eating Out . . .

As in every part of their lives, Pitta people appreciate quality and good value. Their most favored restaurants are clean, well organized, visually appealing, prompt in service with great food at fair prices.

Japanese (not too oily or salty), Chinese, middle eastern restaurants are good choices. Avoid Mexican, Italian, and even most Indian restaurants as the food is often made too spicy or salty.

DIET for KAPHA

General Considerations

• Changing old patterns to eat less in quantity and frequency but maintaining a high quality of foods is key for balancing Kapha dosha.

• Take low salt, low fat, high fiber, lightly cooked foods.

• Kapha people are the only ones who can happily skip breakfast. Eating between 10AM and 6PM is best.

• Take a gentle walk after eating. Avoid sleeping after meals as this adds to heaviness in the body.

• Fast one day a week.

• Be mindful not to use food for emotional support. This will definitely cause weight gain (especially consuming chocolate and late night ice cream).

• Kapha is increased in early morning, later in the evening, and in the spring. Be most careful with your diet at these times, avoiding heavy breakfasts or late night kitchen raids.

• Qualities of food that balance Kapha are pungent, light, dry, astringent, bitter, and hot. Take proportionately more of these and more often.

• Qualities of food that unbalance Kapha are sweet, heavy, sour, oily, salty, and cold. Take less of these and less frequently.

Daily Eating Routines for Kapha Types

• Best to eat twice a day at midday and in early evening with at least a 5-6 hour gap between meals.

• Take only juice or tea for breakfast.

• Take 3-4 servings of whole grains, plus . . .
  2 servings of high quality low fat, protein rich foods.
  4-5 servings of fresh vegetables.
  1 serving of fruit.

Drink only when thirsty.
Eat only when hungry.

Shopping List for Kapha
(reduce and/or copy and take one when you shop
and place one on the refrigerator)
* means occasionally

GRAINS: amaranth, barley, buckwheat, corn, millet, quinoa, basmati rice, rice cakes

LEGUMES: aduki, black beans, black-eye peas, garbanzos, limas, navy beans, navy, pinto, red lentil, split peas, white peas

ANIMAL FOODS: chicken and turkey (dark meat), eggs, wild game

DAIRY: ghee, goat milk, lassi

VEGETABLES: asparagus, beets, beet greens, bell pepper, broccoli, brussels sprouts, burdock, cabbage, carrot, cauliflower, celery, corn, daikon, green beans, jicama, kohlrabi, leafy greens, leeks, lettuce, mushrooms, okra, onion, parsley, peas, radish, spinach, sprouts, summer squash, turnips, watercress

NUT and SEEDS: *pumpkin, *sunflower

FRUITS: apple, apricots, berries, cherries, cranberries, dry figs, mango, peaches, pears, persimmon, pomegranate, prune, quince, raisin, *strawberries

SWEETENERS: raw honey, fruit juice concentrate

OILS: mustard seed, *almond, *corn, *sunflower

CONDIMENTS and SPICES: black pepper, chili, coriander leaf (cilantro), garlic, ginger, mustard, mint leaves, and all spices, generally, with the exception of tamarind

DRINKS: aloe vera juice, fruit and vegetable juice, grain coffee (Pero, Caffix), *coffee, *black tea, spiced herbal teas

Preparation Tips for Kapha Diets

GRAINS: Small portions are helpful to satisfy and sustain energy.

Fruit sweetened granolas, grain flakes, puffed grains, and crisp breads are best.

LEGUMES: Beans are important as they are the best low fat protein source. Cook as described in the Vata section.

MEATS: Generally should be of light quality and cooked with herbs and spices to facilitate fat absorption.

DAIRY: Most dairy food is too heavy and cooling. A little ghee can help with digestion. Kapha lassi can be taken in moderation (1 part low fat yoghurt to 3-4 parts warm water, honey, black pepper, and ginger)

VEGETABLES: All vegetables that grow above the ground are good. Roots are a little too earthy for regular use. Raw or lightly steamed vegetables are best.

FRUITS: Fruits that are not too sweet, sour, or juicy are best. Dried fruit is a great snack or travel food.

OILS: Use sparingly, substituting water cooking where possible.

SWEETENERS: Honey is best. Use no more than one tablespoon per day. Never heat or cook with honey. According to Ayurveda, honey becomes toxic to the body once heated.

SPICES: Use very little salt or use salt substitutes. Use of herbs and spices to stimulate the palate is very useful.

DRINKS: Kapha people can take a little black tea or coffee occasionally. Use a little ginger in black tea and nutmeg or cardamon with coffee. If these don't agree with you, try spiced cider or hot lemon and honey to start your day. Drink only when thirsty and only enough to stop thirst.

When Eating Out . . .
- Order salads rather than soup.
- Take hot water rather than ice water.
- Enjoy salad bars, Mexican (non-dairy dishes), Indian, Chinese, Thai, and vegetarian restaurants.
- Take a light wine with meals or a cocktail to start.

To help integrate all of the information in this section, I have provided sample menus. The suggestions here are not intended to exhaust what is possible, but to provide simple, somewhat generic ideas that I hope are useful. As most people cannot eat their main meal at lunch time, the dinner menus are more extensive.

Sample Menus for Vata Dosha

	Warm Weather	Cold Weather
BREAKFAST:	cool, creamy rice pudding with hot spicy tea	hot wholegrain cereal with hot milk or soymilk, applesauce with cinnamon, and hot ginger tea
LUNCH:	red lentil dahl with omelette, fresh cilantro and sliced lime, chapati and chutney, steamed young mustard greens, cool herb tea	French onion soup, with tofu brown rice and chutney, steamed carrot and asparagus, hot spicy tea
DINNER:	avocado appetizer, oriental-style noodle salad with tofu or poultry, whole grain cookies, ginger tea	vegetable stew, baked chicken or spicy aduki beans, basmati and wild rice, kale with a little ghee, fruit tart, chamomile tea
SNACK:	fresh seasonal fruits, vegetable juices	energy bars, whole grain cookies, crackers with soft cheese, fresh-roasted nuts, hot drinks

Sample Menu for Pitta Dosha

	Warm Weather	**Cool Weather**
BREAKFAST:	whole grain granola or muesli with milk or soy milk, herb tea	oatmeal with hot milk and almond slivers, dates or raisins, hot apple cider
LUNCH:	large green salad with light oil and lemon dressing, whole grain crackers and soft cheese or vegetable pate	vegetable, bean, and barley soup, chapati, and steamed greens
DINNER:	bean burger or grilled chicken, marinated vegetables, herbed rice, fruit pie, herb tea	baked beans, whole wheat muffins, steamed vegetable medley, date bar, grain coffee
SNACK:	fresh fruit	roasted pumpkin or sunflower seeds

Sample Menu for Kapha Dosha

	Warm Weather	**Cool Weather**
BREAKFAST:	fresh fruit, cold cereal with goat or soy milk, mint tea	hot cornmeal cereal and dried apricots with ginger, licorice tea
LUNCH:	bean salad, fresh green salad, rye crackers, lemon grass tea	vegetable soup, rice cakes
DINNER:	Quinoa or millet grain salad, sauteed tofu and steamed vegetables, green salad	baked beans, cornbread, steamed greens and onions, apple crisp, grain coffee

SNACKS: fresh fruit or vegetables   popcorn, sunflower or
                                                pumpkin seeds, corn
                                                chips

The Ayurvedic Cookbook, by Amadea Morningstar gives more menu suggestions for all seasons and circumstances specific to dosha dominance. Her book is a wealth of information in all aspects of food and food preparation from the Ayurvedic point of view. Her recipes are all vegetarian, easy, interesting, and varied in style. Whole food, macrobiotic, and ethnic recipe books are other useful sources for recipes, planning, etc. Chinese, Thai, and French cooking styles are particularly good for meat recipes as they use spice and herbs so well.

AGNI—The Fire of Beauty

Unique to Ayurveda is the concept of agni. Most simply put, agni is digestive fire: the power to convert what isn't you—i.e. food, drinks, sights, sounds, feelings, information—into what is you (your body, emotions, and intelligence). It is agni that has the power to digest food well, making all nutrients available to the tissues. It is agni that powers the mind to be intelligently disciplined to achieve inner beauty. It is agni that also cleans toxins and excess wastes from the system, keeping the digestive tract clean and the outer body fresh and glowing. So, of course, strong, healthy, balanced agni is necessary to keep the body and mind balanced and beautiful.

More usually than not, problems come to the surface for us psychologically and physically when agni is low or too high. Agni that is too low will be the cause of poor digestion of what we take in. When agni is too high, however, it will literally burn foods up before they can be assimilated.

Signs of low agni are:

gas	difficulty waking
burping	scanty or no perspiration
slow digestion	constipation
tired mind	dull complexion

Signs of high agni are:

strong belching	excessive talking
heavy perspiration	burning sensations in
rashes	digestive tract
diarrhea	irritability and anger
hyper-excitablity	

Guidelines for Balancing Agni . . .

To improve Agni:
• Eat smaller meals.
• Sip lime or lemon water.
• Sip warm ginger tea (Recipe: take a pinch of dry ginger and simmer in 1 cup of water until a quarter of the water is boiled away or steep a few slices of fresh ginger in hot water. Drink a little before and a little after your meal). A small amount of ginger tea sweetened with maple syrup before a meal is particularly good for Pitta types.
• Take a pinch of trikatu before meals (made of equal amounts of ginger, black pepper and cayenne, a pinch of which is sprinkled onto a quarter teaspoon of honey). This is especially good for Kapha types.
• Vata types can take a pinch of fresh ginger root that has been chopped finely and mixed with a little salt before a meal.
• Chewing is very important. Chew your food until it is at least liquidy before you swallow.
• Sip warm water with your meals.
• A little umeboshi plum or small amount of melted ghee on grains can help Vata types.

• Gentian bitters and fresh cilantro or parsley with a little black pepper can help agni for Pitta types.

• Light diet and pungent spices can help improve the agni in Kapha types.

• Agni can also be improved by fasting and herbal medications. These procedures should be done with the guidance of an Ayurvedic health care practitioner.

• If there is a lot of toxic build-up in the body and digestion is very weak, hydrochloric acid tablets and/or digestive enzymes may be used for a short period of time until there is a general improvement in health. Once again, take such advice only from a holistically minded physician or dietician.

• Some naturally occurring digestive enzymes can be made available by swallowing more saliva before you eat. This is particularly helpful in the digestion of carbohydrates. To bring more saliva to the mouth, run the tongue between the teeth and lips in a clockwise, then anticlockwise direction while keeping the mouth closed.

• Digestion is best when the right nostril is open and clear. To help open the nostril if its blocked or congested, press the fist of the left hand up into the right arm pit, resting the right arm over the fist. At the same time, press the left nostril closed with your right middle finger. Hold this position for a few minutes until you feel the right nostril begin to clear. This is not necessarily specifically to increase agni, but is an excellent technique to aid digestion. Do this before eating.

• Mudra (Hand Gesture) for Improving Agni:

Sit cross-legged or on a chair with your back straight. Rest your hands, palms upwards on your knees. Join the middle finger and thumbs of each hand. Rest this way a few minutes before meals, breathing calmly and giving thanks for the food you are about to eat.

To reduce Agni:
• follow Pitta diet
• find constructive ways to release anger, frustration, and outrage
• drink a tea of equal amounts of cumin, coriander, fennel seed

How An Ayurvedic Diet Will Keep Your Body Beautiful
Ayurvedic diet is . . .
• high in whole grains and other fiber-rich foods that provide lasting energy throughout the day. Fiber helps maintain a toned digestive tract by providing bulk which helps toxins and excesses to be evacuated. When the intestines are regularly cleaned, the body does not become overloaded with undigested material that would otherwise seek elimination through the skin.
• low in fat, helping to keep the blood clean and prevent a clogging up of veins, arteries, and organs, commonly associated with a diet rich in saturated fats. Good circulation and the circulatory system works efficiently to cleanse and nourish the whole system, and naturally helps weight control.
• low in refined sugars that are empty calories which only serve to pack on the weight. Refined carbohydrates give the body a quick boost of energy that is always followed by a physical (and emotional) low. This stresses the pancreas and adrenals, devitalizing the body. Refined carbohydrates deplete the body of minerals which are so important for all vital functions. It is the combination of refined carbohydrates and excess protein which forces toxins to the skin surface in the form of pimples.
• high in minerals that keep the body looking alive and charged with energy. Minerals greatly contribute to that intangible radiant, fresh, and magnetic look of a person in good health.

• low in animal proteins, yet rich in vegetable proteins. Low protein diets weaken the body and cause a hollow, sunken look to the face. Diets high in animal proteins increase the toxicity of waste products in the body due to their slow transit time (It takes meat about three days to completely be digested and leave the system.) This slows digestion and depletes the body of minerals. Vegetable proteins, on the other hand, fully nourish the body, being quickly and efficiently metabolized. At the same time, not everyone will want to or feel good with being vegetarian. Thus, Ayurveda has the means of making meats more digestible with such spices as garlic, ginger, cumin, cayenne, and black pepper.

• low in salt. Diets high in salt tend to make the mind and body stiff and tight. Having a constricting influence on the body, it tends to slow circulation and create a retention of fluid. This can create that sunken effect under the eyes and make someone look puffy. In Ayurveda, a very low salt diet is suggested whenever there are skin problems.

• devoid of strong stimulants or depressives such as coffee, sodas, or alcohol. These stress the body's organs and make skin loose and flabby, furrowing the brow and producing bags under the eyes in the long run.

• high in fresh organic foods whenever possible. These are nutritionally the richest, coming from healthy soil and thus carry the strongest, vital energy. This contributes to a radiant, rich glow in our face and skin in general.

SUPPLEMENTATION

Ayurvedic diet is based on age-old dietary practices which have been proven to produce healthy, happy people and stable cultures. We have listed and explained why foods such as whole grains, legumes, vegetables, and spices are used the way they are.

At the same time, the picture of modern civilization is very different from the one that existed when the great Ayurvedic treatises were written. Today, most of our foods are produced by large agribusinesses which use methods that deplete the soil, pollute the water, and produce foods low in nutrients. Hybridization, forced growing methods, and high quantities of fertilizers help these businesses to produce crops with a high profit margin, but leave us wanting for sustenance. This is why we are the best fed, but possibly the most poorly nourished generation in the history of the world. Even foods that one finds on the Ayurvedic food lists can be low in nutrition, not because they are inherently this way, but because modern technology has rendered them so. Thus, one could be eating correctly, in terms of one's dosha dominance and circumstances, and still not be getting proper nourishment. This is also aggravated when agni is poor or variable. Encouraging the use of organic foods will help this. But, such foods are currently not that abundant in the marketplace. We also have to deal with poor quality water, air and soil. Depleted soil will make even organic foods lacking in vital trace minerals. Modern researchers are discovering that insufficient levels of trace nutrients in our diet heightens the risk of getting various degenerative diseases common in this day and age. It is also a fact that such trace elements are essential for healthy skin, hair, and nails. So, what is the answer? Or—on a personal note—what more can we do to strengthen ourselves?

The concept of supplementation is not unfamiliar to Ayurveda. However, when taking an herbal compound or concentrated foodstuff as a supplement to one's diet, several problems identified by Ayurvedic theory need to be addressed. As many people today have turned to supplementation, these observations are particularly helpful in making sound choices.

1) If the system is not thoroughly clean from ama, supplements can go undigested. They may not only be of little use, but may actually increase the toxicity of the body. Instead, Ayurveda uses rejuvenatives, or "rasayanas."

Rasayanas are traditionally given when the body has been thoroughly cleansed internally so that concentrated doses of nutrients can get straight to the tissues that need them. These Ayurvedic "superfoods" and herbal preparations are used for their exceptionally high nutritional content. One of the most popular and common is *Chywan-prash*, which contains amla fruit—exceptionally high in Vitamin C. However, again, supplementation of this kind is not considered beneficial if there are blockages or toxins in the system. They will not be digested well and may, as a result, even add to the problem.

2) Supplements may be refined parts of natural substances or totally artificial. The body is not always able to use them thoroughly. Not being from the natural world of food substances they either do not register as nutrients to the body or may need large supplies of other nutrients to metabolize them thoroughly. This may lead to deficiency in other nutritional areas; a robbing Paul to pay Peter situation. In this case, it is best to chose supplements that are as close to natural as possible. The more synthetic they are, the more they will aggravate Pitta dosha. Along with being as natural as possible, it is important to match supplements to one's dosha dominance. For example, Vitamin E capsules are better for Vata people than would be Vitamin E in a chalky tablet form. Blue-green algae seems to be helpful to Vata and Kapha types, but not so much for Pitta types. Thus, one should make every attempt to ensure that supplementation does not disturb the doshas. This is best done if one consults a trained Ayurvedic physician or dietician versed in Ayurveda.

3) Many of the supplements known in the west are not known in the east and vice versa. Many of the Ayurvedic preparations used to assist and rejuvenate the body may not be readily available here in the west. It, therefore, becomes necessary to study and understand what is available here in Ayurvedic terms. Some of the best supplements available are "superfoods" such as spirulina, blue-green algae, young grain powders, and sea vegetable tablets. Each one of these products has their specific action on the body and, therefore, influences or favors certain doshas more.

4) Although supplementation is one way of ensuring that the body gets the nutrition it needs, Ayurveda also has herbs that may not con-

tain the needed nutrient, but can help the body to assimilate better, hence getting the nutrients out of the diet. This is a medical issue and requires the mastery of an Ayurvedic healer to be able to properly prescribe such.

5) A major problem with supplementation is that when the supplement is discontinued, so is the benefit. Ayurveda ideally seeks to improve assimilation as well as the standard diet to fulfill all needs.

Supplementation is a tricky business and is best done with professional help. It should never be considered a substitute for sound diet, environmental awareness, and stress management techniques.

What about Vitamins and Minerals?

Although classical Ayurveda does not teach about the importance of vitamins and minerals, I have included a list of beauty-related problems that can arise when certain vitamins and minerals are missing and in what foods they can be found to make up for deficiencies. Remember, a varied, healthy diet is most crucial to maintaining a vibrant appearance.

VIT./MIN.	SIGN of DEFICIENCY	FOUND IN . . .
Vit. A (strong Pitta need)	dry, rough, scaly skin, wrinkling, itching, pimples, loss of elasticity, premature aging, enlarged pores, irregular sebaceous gland production, dandruff, split/ peeling nails, poor night-vision, burning & itching eyes, thickening of cornea, skin slow to heal and grow	dark green and orange vegetables, corn, soy, lentils, garbanzo beans, miso, butter, liver, crab, eggs, fish oil, whole milk
Vit. B1	poor digestion, fatigue,	whole grains, molasses,

VIT./MIN.	SIGN of DEFICIENCY	FOUND IN . . .
Thiamine	stress, alcoholism, premature aging	green vegetables, brewer's yeast, beans
Vit. B2 Riboflavin	wrinkling around lips, oily 'T' zone, tiny black heads on nose, small white heads, scaly nose and forehead, cracks around lips and eyes, bloodshot eyes that itch and burn, light sensitivity, hair loss, premature aging	millet, corn, soy, whole wheat, rye, wheat germ, almonds, beans, milk, avocado, nuts, blackstrap molasses, dark greens, organic meats, egg yolk, nori, wakame, brewer's yeast
Vit. B3 Niacin (strong need for Vata)	poor circulation, low metabolism of fats and carbohydrates, dryness, inflammation, fatigue, bad breath, abnormal skin pigmentation	wheat, buckwheat, barley, wild rice, black beans, almonds, peanuts & other nuts, sesame seeds, seafood, dark greens, shitake mushrooms, lean meat, milk, rice bran
Vit. B5 Pantothenic Acid	stress related skin eruptions, hair loss, wrinkles, premature aging, allergies	whole grains, poultry, corn, beans, broccoli, cabbage, cauliflower, sunflower seeds, vegetable oils, organ meats, egg yolks, salmon
Vit. B6 Pyroxidine (strong need for Kapha)	poor digestion, hormonal imbalance, slow healing of skin, eczema, water retention, PMS, dry or oily rashy skin, dandruff,	brown rice, buckwheat, beans, carrots, cabbage, sunflower seeds, peanuts, fish, organ meats, lean meats, brewer's yeast, blackstrap molasses,

	stretch marks, wrinkles around mouth, thinning hair, premature aging	bananas, wheat germ
Vit. B9 Folic Acid	anemia, sallow skin, gray or brown skin discoloration, hangnails, hair loss, dull hair	whole grains, salad and green vegetables, wheat germ, brewer's yeast, mushrooms, oysters, milk, salmon, bran, sprouted grains, organ meats, soy products, naturally fermented pickles, yoghurt, nori, spirulina
Vit. B12	premature aging, fatigue, insomnia, poor concentration and memory, aggression	whole grain, liver, milk, oysters, salmon, naturally fermented pickles, tamari, unpasteurized miso
BIOTIN	grayish skin, anemia, depression, poor fat metabolism, dermatitis, balding	liver, brown rice, and other whole grains, eggs, fish, nuts, legumes, liver, cauliflower
CHOLINE	fat accumulation, poor immunity, weak nerves, premature grey hair	lecithin, brewer's yeast, liver
INOSITOL	eczema, hair loss, high cholesterol, constipation, fat build-up	lecithin, blackstrap molasses, brown rice, barley, oats, legumes, beef heart, seeds
PABA	nervousness, fatigue, digestive problems,	liver, eggs, brown rice, wheat germ, blackstrap

VIT./MIN.	SIGN of DEFICIENCY	FOUND IN . . .
	premature greying and wrinkles, vitiligo	molasses
Vit. C	(Warning: high amounts of Vit. C can be problematic for Pitta types).	
	poor skin tone, bruises easily, thread veins, wrinkles, premature aging, cellulite, weak hair roots	asparagus, alfalfa sprouts, cabbage family, mustard greens, peas, okra, red and green peppers, mung beans, tomatoes, berries, citrus fruits, melons, mangoes, papayas, pineapples, organ meats, fish, eggs, dairy products
BIOFLAVINOIDS		
	weak walls of blood vessels, thread veins, varicose veins, bleading gums, bruising, eczema	Same products as Vit. C
Vit. D (strong need for Kapha)	weak teeth, bones, hair, and nails	sunlight, fish oils, flax oil, dried fish, whole grains, dark greens, eggs, salmon, sardines, herring, butter, eggs
Vit. E	premature aging, low sex drive, rough and dry and tired skin, poor muscle tone, dryness, varicose veins, scars	wheat germ, whole grains, dark greens, nuts & seeds, cold-pressed vegetable oils, liver, butter, milk, eggs, organ meats, molasses

Essential Fatty Acids	brittle and lusterless hair, eczema, dry skin, nail problems, dandruff, allergies	wheat germ, Omega 3 oil, flax seeds, lecithin, cod liver oil
Vit. K	low energy in cells, premature aging	yoghurt, eggs, blackstrap molasses, milk, fish oil
Calcium	weak hair, teeth, & nails, PMS, insomnia	sea vegetables, dark greens, sesame seeds, sunflower seeds, eggs, milk, cheese, nuts, dried fruit, sardines, shell fish
Copper	loss of hair color, poor skin tone	organ meats, eggs, poultry, kelp, whole-grains, liver, seafood
Iodine	thyroid dysfunction, dry & wrinkled skin	kelp, onions, beans, seafood
Iron	pale, lusterless skin and nails, poor vitality, brittle hair, weak nails, thinning hair, itching skin	egg yolk, leafy greens, parsley, dulse, nettle tea, whole grains, miso, tekka, molasses, raisins, pumpkin seeds, nuts, berries, increase of exercise
Magnesium	stress-related skin problems, low vitality, low muscle tone, low calcium & Vit. C metabolism, tense muscles, irritability, psoriasis	seafood, wholegrains, yellow corn, dulse, soy products, lentils, dried fruits, nuts, leafy greens, apples, celery, lemon, figs, grapefruit

VIT./MIN.	SIGN of DEFICIENCY	FOUND IN . . .
Phosphorus	bone loss, muscle weakness, fatigue	whole grains, beans, nuts, vegetables, lean meats, sunflower seeds
Potassium	muscular weakness, poor digestion, dry skin, acne, dermatitis	bananas, watercress, sea vegetables, green peppers, dried fruits
Selenium	premature aging, loss of skin elasticity, dandruff	eggs, whole grains, beans, onion, tomatoes, tuna, garlic, liver
Silica	flabbiness, weak nails, dull hair	horsetail herb
Sulphur	scaly skin, eczema, brittle lusterless hair, weak nails	fish, eggs, nuts, cabbage family, apples, cranberries, beans, onions, watercress, kale, currants
Zinc	loss of skin elasticity, wrinkles, stretch marks, white spots on nails, hair loss	pumpkin and sunflower seeds, seafood, organ meats, mushrooms, eggs, wheat germ

Generally speaking, if one eats a good quality, organically grown Ayurvedic diet appropriate to one's dosha dominance and has strong agni, most of these vitamins and minerals will be found in what you eat daily. Vitamin and mineral supplementation becomes more essential if you have a diet that is high in red meat, refined carbohydrates and sugar. Thus, such a diet is worth avoiding.

At the same time, because of the environmental factors mentioned, there may be various deficiencies, in which case supplementation beyond food sources may be necessary. As regards beauty, many vitamin companies are coming out with herbal supplements specifically for hair, nails, and skin. Please refer to the Source Appendix.

Fasting *(Kshud)*

Fasting over long periods of time is strongly frowned upon in the Ayurvedic tradition. It is felt that long term deprivation eventually will lead to over-indulgence. The body feels its life force threatened by being deprived of food and then wants to stock up again. So rather than have the desired cleansing effect, such fasting produces fear which leads to an overloading of the system. There are two exceptions to this view in Ayurveda. The first is, when due to illness, a person has no appetite. In such circumstances, soft grains are recommended as a way of reintroducing food to the system once hunger has returned. The second situation is in purification therapy under the guidance of an Ayurvedic physician or practitioner when other cleansing methods, such as Pancha Karma, are not available.

Short-term fasts of one to three days, however, done on a regular weekly or bi-monthly basis are considered very beneficial. They give the digestive system time to rest and recuperate without starving the tissues or evoking adverse emotional reactions.

When Vata is high, fasting on warm water only is useful for a day at a time and no more than twice a month. Adding a little honey and lemon juice to maintain energy. A water fast for longer periods severely weakens the body and can take a long time to fully recover. Longer fasting for Vata conditions can be accomplished by selecting a cleansing, yet nutrifying, mono-diet such as kichadi. Such a mono-diet can be followed for up to a month.

Amadea Morningstar has over ten interesting kichadi recipes in her book, *The Ayurvedic Cookbook*. The following recipe is specifically given for improving digestion. It takes ninety minutes to prepare and makes three to four servings. If using it for fasting purposes, make it fresh every day so that the energetic quality in the food is strong and the nutrients fresh and full.

Amadea's Digestive Kichadi

½ teaspoon cumin seed
2 Tablespoons ghee or sunflower oil
3 bay leaves
1 teaspoon coriander seed
½ teaspoon tumeric powder
1 teaspoon dry oregano
½ teaspoon sea salt
1 three-inch strip of kombu sea vegetable
1 teaspoon grated, fresh ginger root
½ cup of basmati rice (washed and drained)
½ cup of split mung dahl (washed and drained)
4-6 cups of water
3 cups of fresh seasonal vegetables (not nightshade family, i.e.
tomatoes, potatoes, peppers, eggplants) diced into ½ inch cubes

Warm the ghee in a sauce pan. Lightly brown the cumin, bay, coriander, and oregano. Stir in turmeric, rice, and dahl. Add water, kombu, and ginger. Simmer covered for 1 hour. Add the vegetables and cook until they and the rice mixture are soft.

Dr. Robert Svoboda offers a very traditional kichadi recipe in his book, *Prakruti, Your Ayurvedic Constitution.* This recipe makes a substantial amount so it would work for at least two people for one day of fasting.

Svoboda's Kichadi

2 cups of basmati rice
1 cup of split mung beans
8-12 cups of water
2 Tablespoons Ghee
1 teaspoon cumin powder
1 teaspoon coriander seed
¼-½ teaspoon tumeric powder
3-5 whole cardamon pods
1-2 teaspoons ginger powder
pinch of salt or powdered kelp
pinch of asafoetida powder (hing)

Dr. Svoboda suggests using less mung beans if you have digestive problems, using 1 part beans to three parts rice. If your digestion is strong and feels the need for more protein, use equal amounts of beans to rice.

Rinse, drain, then soak the rice and mung beans separately for one half hour. After soaking, rinse and drain again. Sauté the powders and seeds in ghee. Add sauteed mixture to water. Add the rice and beans to water, then ginger, salt or kelp, and cardamon pods. Cover and simmer until both beans and rice are soft (approximately one hour).

Water fasts are only useful for very short periods when Pitta is high, too. Fruit and vegetable juices, in sufficient quantity to satisfy hunger, will work well here. Suitable juices include apple, pear, white grape, prune, pomegranate, celery, cucumber, and juices from greens.

When Kapha is high, water fasting is ideal and if done one day a week it helps stimulate an otherwise sluggish tendency in the digestive process. Apple, cranberry, cherry, and pomegranate juices are also useful for fasting when Kapha is in excess.

Sometimes due to a lack of fiber in juices, constipation becomes a problem. In this case, use a natural bulk laxative like psyllium seed husk or linseed (flax) mixed with juice or—in the case where one is on a fast using one of the Kichadi recipes—mix with water. Half a teaspoon of Triphala (a common Ayurvedic herbal mixture) that has been soaked a few hours in warm water, taken at bedtime, also works as a gentle laxative. It has the added benefit of balancing the doshas and purifying the digestive tract.

WORKING WITH LIFESTYLE

"The whole world is a teacher for the wise and
for the fool the whole universe is full of enemies."
Charaka

Ayurveda teaches that beauty, health, and a full, happy, long life are achievable only by understanding how all aspects of life contribute to bringing balance to the body and mind. There are many guidelines given in the classic texts but ultimately this information is useful only if it becomes part of your daily life. Routines provided in these texts should be adopted, not because they are ultimate truths—more real or true than much other advice, or even just because they feel good—but because they work. Getting results is the best incentive for developing the self-discipline necessary to maintain such practices and to radiate health and beauty. As Charaka says, use your life experience, coupled with the knowledge of Ayurveda, as your teacher to create a world that is a nurturing friend rather than an aggravating enemy. This chapter provides information about many aspects of daily life. Read it, try it, adopt what works, making changes gradually as they begin to make sense for you. Remember that ultimately all the factors that help establish positive health for the body and mind definitely contribute to a beautiful body and magnetic personality.

GRACEFUL WORK LIFE
Most of us spend at least a third of our lives and most of our waking hours involved in a work situation. The work we choose, the environment that puts us in, the physical, emotional and spiritual demands that are placed on us in this situation, definitely impact the internal balance of the doshas—which directly influence how we

66

look and feel.

People are attracted to jobs because of their personal interest, individual inclinations, inherent skills, or a combination of one or more of these aspects. A great deal of this attraction is influenced by their constitutional types. As with all choices they are not necessarily most balancing to the doshas, but can be modified to be more so. Working gracefully, then, relies upon learning how to satisfy natural desires and aspirations without diminishing one's performance by creating body imbalances. Simply learning how you can keep yourself together to be able to do your best, helps you to get where you want to, in the way you like to do it.

For each constitutional type there are ways of working that feel natural and satisfying. However, without a skillful handling of natural work tendencies, they can get out of hand and then become detrimental to the mind and body in the long run. As energy becomes less than optimal and distraction increases, the body and mind experience more suffering. In this case, experiencing and radiating beauty become less and less possible. So, let's examine the inclinations of each body type and how to best maintain energy in the work situation.

Vata people are attracted to work that is exciting, unpredictable, intense, varied, creative; work that involves travel, sensitivity, and in an environment where they work with a lot of people, ideas, moods, and sensations. Too many of these factors are Vata increasing and will eventually cause Vata imbalance. Environments and circumstances that directly have a negative influence on Vata types are those that are cold, drafty, dusty, noisy, chaotic, and where there are a lot of electronic stimuli and wiring, such as computers, copiers, phone lines, fluorescent lighting, etc.

There is no problem in pursuing a job that is Vata-genic if you are prepared to take time to tame the imbalances it produces. If you feel that you don't have such time, your body will force the issue by being sick for periods of time.

To help keep Vata in balance as much as possible:
- Create flexible routines.
- Take periods of rest and relaxation after periods of intense work.
- Treat yourself to an oily, aromatherapy massage periodically.
- Go to a quiet park or a walk in the country as often as possible.
- Dress for warmth and comfort.
- Wear earplugs if you are in an environment where there is excessive noise.
- Eat regularly.
- Get to bed early as often as possible.
- Avoid making decisions at high Vata times, such as early mornings or late afternoons. As much as possible, do not schedule important meetings at these times, as these are not your clearest times of day.
- Avoid unnecessary travel. If you have to travel, try to include some nurturing and pleasant activity during the trip or for when you get back.
- Delegate as much as possible and try not to take your work home.
- Avoid the tendency to keep changing jobs for the sake of variety.

Pitta types are practical, preferring to work with the concrete, such as numbers, schedules, production of something, buying or selling—something they can feel passionate about, take risks in, and have opportunities for innovation and competition. Being leaders in whatever the field they are in, they must be wary of their compulsive tendencies. To help them to balance, Pitta types should:
- Avoid becoming too intense or single-minded in your work life.
- Build a strong work team around you so that you don't keep on over-stretching yourself.
- If possible, work in your own business.
- Work on anger and frustration that quickly arises when delays or incompetence is encountered.
- Avoid contact with industrial chemicals.
- Avoid having to work in intense heat, light, or sunshine for long periods of time.
- Avoid lunchtime meetings as your mood will be the least appeal-

ing and productive if you are hungry.
• Develop a loving, calm home life with family and/or circle of friends.
• Take regular visits to a health club to reduce stress.
• Meditate to create space in your life.
• Practice skilled relaxation to help the body keep pace with your active mind and work hard—play hard mentality.
• Take cold showers.

The steady, stable, conscientious, loving nature of Kapha lends itself to work as great administrators, receptionists, accountants, counselors and other "caring" professions. They have no problem with routine or repetitive tasks. While their natural stamina and consistency make them a reliable member of a work team, to help maintain their balance in the work place Kapha types should:
• bring challenge into their work life to combat monotony.
• include physical activity in their work, i.e., take a walk after lunch. Exercise and fresh air will increase their alertness in the afternoon.
• eat lightly at lunch time. Avoid sweet snacks at coffee breaks.
• take advantage of their great memory capacity. Stay involved with learning new things, whether they be job related or otherwise. Such stimulation will keep them moving forward in their career.
• set goals. They will then be able to effortlessly make steady advances and even accumulate wealth if they keep their focus.
• be true to their spiritual nature, but do not get too overly involved with the problems of others.

CLIMATE CONSIDERATIONS
Climate is a major factor in influencing the body's balance. Many of us cannot choose exactly where we live for any number of reasons. We can, however, choose wisely where we go for vacations or periods of rest and rejuvenation.

Vata types feel best in warm, moist climates, preferably near the ocean, a swimming pool, lake or river so the heat can be enjoyed without it becoming too intense. Most Vata people love the sun. They are better off sunbathing with a cool drink than hiking in the sun all day. Lovers of intensity, they should make the focus of their vacations and breaks rest as well as play. Climates such as those found in Florida, Hawaii, the South Sea Islands, the Mediterranean coastline and the tropics are preferable.

Pitta types hate to be overheated, so cool, breezy, drier climates are best. Being near water—rivers, lakes, oceans—and places that are lush and green are most nourishing. Ireland, Sweden, Norway, the Pacific Northwest spring to mind. (Interestingly, these areas are associated with Pitta physique, flaming red heads with freckles, tall blondes, and lumberjacks!) They should choose places with plenty to do; places of interest to visit in the daytime, quality restaurants, elegant nightlife, and gentle physical challenges.

Kapha types are most comfortable with dry, warm, even fairly hot climates—as long as they can take siestas. They enjoy the slow pace of southern or Mediterranean life. Turkey, the Greek Islands, or Southwestern States of the United States are ideal. Southern cuisine offers just enough garlic and chili and not too much cheese and tahini! Some organized activity is helpful as Kaphas are too happy just sitting around. They suffer most in heavy, humid weather.

Chronic mental and physical problems may develop if one lives in a climate that most exacerbates one's constitutional type. In such cases, you may consider relocation. If this is out of the question, one should make attempts to manipulate one's home micro-climate to improve your quality of life. Vata types benefit from open, cozy fires, humidifiers, central heating, and window double glazing to prevent draughts and to create a warm, secure climactic atmosphere. Pitta types need ceiling fans, windows that can be readily opened, even air conditioning, so long as it is regulated so as to not create too great a contrast with the outside environment. Kapha types need dry warmth. In cold weather, forced air heat is excellent and air conditioning in intense heat.

Become aware of the kind of climate that suits you best. The more comfortable you feel in your body, the more you will be able to project both your inner and outer beauty.

MASSAGE

Everyone needs massage on a regular basis whether you do it for yourself, enjoy one with a partner, or get one from a professional masseuse. In just the same way as a machine needs greasing, the body loves to be oiled for sheer pleasure as well as to protect it against the ravages of time.

Vata people—in particular—should give themselves an oily massage daily; in the early morning or before a warm bath in the evening. Regular professional massage at least monthly is advised as Vata types need to be cared for to feel secure. Vata types are dry and cool by nature, so benefit greatly from the nurturing quality of a warm oil massage. This kind of oily massage lubricates dry skin, protects joints, provides grounding, and protects Vata dosha from subtle, harmful energies (including radiation and negative emotions) by strengthening the aura.

Vata people are very sensitive to touch. If they can learn to trust someone else, it is one of the ways they can experience love, nurturing and support. Ayurvedic and Swedish styles of massage are best. Rolfing and other forms of deep-tissue massage should be done rarely or only as needed, and with great care as Vata energy is easily disrupted. Even the more subtle energy types of massage can have dramatic effects as Vata types are so sensitive.

For Vata types, oil used should always be warm when applied so it can penetrate more deeply and calm the nervous system. Too much oil may cause disturbances in the Vata's sensitive digestive tract. Suitable oils are sesame, almond, or olive. Herbs such as ashwagandha, shatavari or bala may be added to the oils to create a tonic effect. Mahanarayan or Narayan oils are also very good, especially if there is stiffness or inflammation in the joints. Essential oils of wintergreen, cinnamon, musk, galangal, or cypress increase the warming effect of the oils. Sandalwood, rose, or jasmine are good for facilitating a calm and grounded state of mind. (Use 20 drops per 2 fluid ounces of oil.)

Pitta people enjoy the qualities of regular massage from a well-practiced, highly knowledgeable, loving massage professional. They are less likely to massage themselves as they tend to undervalue self care. Scheduling time to receive massage as a means of providing deep rest and relaxation is very important in balancing the intensity most Pitta people enjoy. Massage with correctly applied oil will enhance the natural lustre of the Pitta's skin, nourish their shapely muscles, and calm their reactive nervous system. Too much oil, and oils that are heating in quality, make Pitta types itchy, thirsty, irritable, even possibly nauseous. Their skin is sensitive and easily becomes rashy or inflamed (This is especially true in hot weather.). Shiatsu, polarity, or other forms of massage that don't use oil, but rather work primarily with the body's electromagnetic field, are also useful for Pittas (and especially called for when there is a high level of skin sensitivity).

Suitable oils should be cooling or neutral in nature. Coconut oil calms and cools the body while reducing thirst and burning sensations. Sunflower oil helps inflamed skin. Olive, sesame, and ghee are more neutral. (If ghee is aged in copper or silver pots it has a more cooling effect.) At times they may be too heating unless cooling herbs or essential oils are added. Herbal oils that are helpful to Pitta include shatavari, gotu kola, bhringaraj, and brahmi. Essential oils that cool the body and the temperament include sandalwood (red, if possible), gardenia, jasmine, rose, honeysuckle, violet, iris, and lotus. Those particularly cooling for the head are sandalwood (often applied to the third eye area), lemon grass, lavender, mint, henna, and vertivert. Pitta people have strong likes and dislikes—and they are prepared to tell their preferences. Some Pittas will like the light, flowery scents, others the fresher smells of mints and lemon, while others go for the more exotic smells of sandalwood, jasmine, and lotus. Follow your intuition and go for your preferences.

Kapha types need massage to improve their circulation and lymph drainage. Their skin and flesh are strong and thick, so can take penetrating massage styles as well as body therapies that shake and pummel the body. Kapha types love to luxuriate in body oils and lotions, but really should use very little as they tend to increase the feeling of heaviness in the body. Using small amounts of hot, sharp, stimulating oils are best, mustard oil being the most commonly recommended. Jojoba oil plus essential oils of sage, cedar, pine, myrrh, musk, patchouli, or cinnamon are also good. Other styles of massage that are useful for Kapha types include shiatsu, Tragering, lymphatic massage, and vigorous Ayurvedic friction massage.

Oils are selected not only by which dosha they benefit, but also according to climate, season, and locale. Castor and sesame oils are good in dry climates because they are heavy and penetrate the skin, going deep into the tissue. Safflower oil is recommended for damp climates where such deep lubricating action is not required. Mustard and sesame are best in cold weather, while coconut and olive are good for hot weather. Oils that can be derived from vegetation that is local to you are considered best in the same way that foods that grow locally help you to maintain balance in your locale.

With increased interest in natural health care and beauty, natural cosmetic oils, not mentioned in the classical Ayurvedic texts, have come onto the market, such as jojoba, grapeseed, avocado, and canola. Jojoba is excellent as it is both light and penetrating. Avocado is rich and nourishing. Canola is a good carrier for essential oils.

In contrast to these natural products is mineral oil. Because oil is a carrier of nutrients into the body, such harsh, poor quality, and unnaturally colored and perfumed oils should never be used on the skin.

To change the heating or cooling effect of any oil to be used, a simple technique is to place oil in red bottles or blue bottles and allow them to stand in the sunlight for about forty days. Oil from red bottles will become more heating in action while those placed in blue bottles will be more cooling.

As many people are of mixed dosha constitution, modifications to what is generally recommended for single dosha types need to be made.

Vata-Pitta types should use less oil than pure Vatas.

Pitta-Kapha types should use sunflower or corn oils.
Vata-Kapha types should use mustard, almond, or olive oil.

Herbal Oils

Prescribing and making herbal oils is the sacred art of an Ayurvedic practitioner specializing in the rejuvenation therapy called Pancha Karma. Many herbs and herbal combinations are used as well as ghee that has been 'washed' or rubbed for long periods of time between copper or silver plates. These processes almost magically transform their base substances into deeply healing medicines. Medicinal herbal oils, known in Sanskrit as Siddha Taila, work primarily on the skin, blood, muscle, connective tissue, lungs, and colon by enhancing metabolic processes in each of these tissues. Herbal oils deeply lubricate and nourish the skin; cleanse and enrich the blood; build and maintain strong muscle and connective tissue; lubricate the joints, keeping them flexible and pain free; and enhance the energy of the lungs and colon which helps to keep skin looking fresh and lustrous.

Several of these oils are now imported, including amla, bhringaraj, mahanarayan, dashmula, guduchi, tulsi, and neem as well as combinations for various conditions and particular dosha dominances. For those interested in making their own herbal oil combinations, what follows are descriptions on how to make oils using traditional methods.

Methods of Preparation—Sesame oil and ghee are most commonly used where extensive healing is needed as they are slow to break down. Coconut and sunflower oils are used when one is wanting to prepare an oil with less heating qualities.

Methods of Preparation

• Mix one part herb with four parts oil and sixteen parts water, e.g. 2 ounces of herb to 4 cups of oil and 16 cups of water. Bring to a boil and simmer until all the water evaporates (approximately 4 to 8 hours). Strain to render the herbal oil.

• Make a strong tea of the desired herbs first, using 2 ounces of herb to 16 cups of water. Strain the decoction and add 4 cups of oil to the liquid. Simmer until all of the water is evaporated.

(In both of the previous methods, one can prevent the oil from scorching by placing a few thin slices of fresh ginger into the oil and tea mixture as it simmers down.)

• Bruise fresh herbs, put them in a jar and cover them with oil. Put them in strong sunlight for 30 days. Strain and keep refrigerated.. (Calendula oil is made this way, using marigold petals.)

• Cayenne, clove, or mustard powder can be simmered directly in oil on a very low flame for several hours.

• Fresh juice of heating herbs like garlic or ginger, or cooling herbs such as comfrey, cilantro, or fennel can be mixed with equal amounts of oil. The oil and juice will separate and spoil, so need refrigeration. Shake well before using. These are not designed to be kept for long periods.

• Add essential oil to a base oil such as jojoba, calendula, almond, grapeseed, or canola; 20 drops of essential oil to 2 fluid ounces of base oil. Always test on a small area of skin to check for allergenic reactions. If this occurs with an oil that you feel good about, dilute more until there is no allergic response.

• Add herbal powders directly to the oil or ghee. This creates a paste that is used more like a body scrub or a cream for points of tension or injury.

Post-Massage Procedures

After you have taken a massage, allow 10 to 20 minutes time to rest and allow the oil to be absorbed. If you are doing self massage, use this time to gently exercise. The excess oil should be removed after this time to avoid your body ingesting the remainder of the oil which often has body toxins in it. Leaving it on will make the body feel heavy, sleepy, lethargic, laxadaisical, possibly even sore. Massage should refresh and invigorate the body and mind. Remove this oil using warmed flour; chickpea for Vata types, barley for Pitta types, and corn or rice for Kapha types. Dust the flour all over the body, rub it in, then rinse it off. An alternative to this dusting is to make a paste with the flour that is applied like a lotion all over the body. Two handfuls of flour and enough water to make the paste is usually sufficient. Once this paste or flour is removed, the skin feels moist, soft, and alive.

EXERCISE *(Vyayama)*
"Dance with the rhythms of life to the harmony of the universe."

Regular exercise is essential to health and vibrant beauty because it helps clear the channels of the body so that all the tissues can be thoroughly cleansed via sweat and other eliminatory channels and be well supplied with nutrients. Exercise is especially helpful for the skin because in order for the skin to renew itself and be fresh and clear, it needs to be cleared of wastes. Exercise also strengthens the body's musculature, keeping it firm and shapely. As explained by our study of the dhatus, strong muscles help support beautiful skin. It builds stamina and boosts heat in the body and the immune response. On a mental/emotional level, exercise helps to reduce tension, reduce anxiety, and promote a sense of overall well being. It also helps one to get deep, restful sleep. Exercise builds mental stamina and provides the energy boost needed to develop and maintain a well-balanced and healthy self-care routine for yourself.

There are many forms of exercise: 1) passive exercise which is done through self-massage or massage by someone else, 2) active exercise which is what we normally think of as exercise (i.e. jogging, team sports, calisthenic-type exercise classes, etc. and 3) energy-balancing type exercises such as yoga, tai chi, and various martial arts exercise processes. Of course, certain types of exercise are recommended for the various constitutional types.

Exercise Guidelines for Vata Types

Vata people love the excitement and feeling of exhilaration that strong exercise brings. They can easily get addicted to this "high," especially as it temporarily slows the mind making the Vata person feel more grounded. Unfortunately, these feelings are short lived as the body becomes more exhausted and the mind speeds up faster than before.

Vata people need to curb their enthusiasm and work slowly to build real strength and stamina. As their bodies tend to be dry, drinking water before, during, and after exercise is a must. Having a high nutrient snack like a sports energy bar or a piece of sweet fruit afterwards is also helpful. Relaxation time after exercise helps calm Vata energy as it helps to recharge and rebalance the body.

Vata people have a tendency toward joint problems and arthritis. Forms of exercise that do not jar the joints are best. Applying warm sesame oil or mustard oil (if joints are arthritic) before active exercise helps protect joints. Wearing elasticated joint supports and good quality supportive and cushioned sports shoes are also good ideas. Generally speaking, exercises that have a smooth rhythm to them are better than chaotic or rough exercise or sports where the flow of energy can become disrupted and injury more likely.

Vata people like change so might want to alternate or switch forms of exercise often. It is best for them to exercise a regular amount at a regular time of day, sticking to one form for a minimum of three weeks at a time. Programs that produce fast results will be more appealing and successful. Good, fast results help maintain a steady discipline so important for grounding the Vata.

Specific Exercise for Vata Types

1) Passive—regular warm oily massage by a loving supportive, calm, and sensitive individual. Learning massage with a friend or lover with a view to massaging each other regularly is great for Vata people who generally need a lot of love and physical reassurance.

2) Active—specific sports include trampolining (or rebounding), swimming, walking, ballet, cross country skiing, low impact aerobics, callanetics, country dancing, ballroom dancing, roller blading/skating, rhythmic workout with weights.

3) Passive and Active—yoga postures, yogic breathing, tai chi chih or various form of tai chi, Taoist energy channeling exercises.

A final note for Vatas is on the use of steam baths and hot tubs. Because these hydrotherapies stimulate circulation and relax and nurture the body they can be quite good for Vatas. However, they can be overdone in which case they may cause the Vata to become more dried out.

Exercise Guidelines for Pitta Types

Pitta people have athletic bodies and strong competitive spirit. They like to drive themselves to the limit, love challenge, and—fortunately or not—have the kind of physical stature that tolerates a lot of abuse. They need to remember to balance their tendency to get overly competitive, intense, and aggressive with allowing themselves to have fun in the midst of their intensity. They need, also, to take periods of relaxation and calm afterwards. Team sports will soften this intensity as well as channel their energies into organization and leadership skills (they generally excel in both). Adventure sports that have a level of danger, competing with the odds or elements are excellent as well.

Pitta people get most easily exhausted and irritable if they either get overheated by over-exercising or by being in too much sunlight. Water sports or sports on snow or ice help to temper the heat. After exercise, a short sauna and a cold plunge will make Pitta types feel great.

Specific Exercises for Pitta Types

1) Passive—self-massage help Pitta people appreciate and pay attention to themselves and their body process. Professional massage should be high quality and precise; satisfy their attentiveness and yet be calming. Shiatsu, Rolfing, Feldenkrais, and sports massage are best.

2) Active—sports can include swimming, skiing, water skiing, wind surfing, hang gliding, aerobics, callanetics, archery, game hunting,

hiking, birdwatching, canoeing, jazz dancing, white water rafting, ballet, horse riding, non-contact martial arts and weapons katars, doubles tennis or squash, and team sports such as water polo, volley ball, basketball, soccer, cricket, hockey, etc.

3) Passive and Active—Hatha Yoga, classic long form tai chi forms, Taoist exercises

Exercise Guidelines for Kapha Types

Of all the body types, people with dominant Kapha qualities are the least naturally inclined toward active exercise. They naturally have strength, endurance, and stamina and, at the same time, cannot see the point in expending energy unless it is absolutely necessary. Exercise is important for Kapha types to help with weight control, stimulate a naturally slow digestive system, improve circulation of lymph, fight cellulite, and provide mental stimulation.

Kapha body types can exercise long and hard without any ill effect, but rarely do. It is better that they find a form of exercise they truly enjoy and will do regularly. Sports that are vigorous and somewhat unpredictable in nature are best, but anything is better than nothing.

Specific Exercises for Kapha Types

1) Passive—deep massage using no or very little oil such as deep-tissue work, shiatsu, or forms of oriental self-inductive Do-In massage that include vigorously tapping of the body.

2) Active—short walks after meals, bowling, various ball sports such as football, basketball, ballroom dancing, horse riding, sledding, belly dancing, playing frisbee, having a pet that needs exercising to stir the Kapha into an act of kindness towards another being in order to do something that they wouldn't do if it were just them.

3) Passive and active—yoga postures, breathing exercises, tai chi chih, Taoist exercises.

It is most important that you enjoy your exercise program and get the results you are seeking. The atmosphere of the exercise space is as important as the type of exercise itself. Keep looking until you find a situation that you find comfortable, supportive, and inspiring. A kind and knowledgeable teacher can be very helpful and inspiring and produce a class atmosphere that promotes faster acquisition of skills than can be gained by books or video tapes. If, however, you cannot find a suitable teacher or class, the books and videos in the Source Appendix at the end of this book are highly recommended.

As a rule, exercise only to half of your capacity. For example, if one hour of tennis exhausts you, play for one-half hour or until you just break a sweat. Exercise less when it is intensely hot or intensely cold to save your energy. Try to breathe evenly when you exercise. This strengthens the lungs and digestive organs, hence improving the color and texture of your skin enormously. Never exercise when you have respiratory disorders, inflammation anywhere in the body, or indigestion. If you have chronic pain, arthritis, joint disorders, or lung problems, seek professional advice and only work with trained instructors. While exercising, wear comfortable clothing made of natural fibers so the skin can 'breathe' and the more subtle forms of energy can flow freely. Be sure to use good quality foot wear to help protect joints for active sports.

Listen to your body. It is good to extend yourself, but don't just blindly push yourself through pain. Be kind and gentle to your body. And above all, whatever you do, enjoy it and make it a natural part of your daily or weekly routine.

Comments on Specific Forms of Exercise

Hatha Yoga Asanas

Yoga postures are ideal to promote beauty on all levels. As physical exercise, it keeps the body supple and youthful as well as improving stamina and strength. It actually relaxes the skin while toning the muscles, giving the body a gentle, yet vital, appearance. Also, many postures help rejuvenate the glandular system, specifically the thyroid, adrenals, and pituitary. All of this helps to reduce stress in the system dramatically and to promote longevity. The precision of the movements demands discipline and concentration, while on the deepest level they can transform emotional states and further one along on one's spiritual path. There are specific postures that help to maintain balance to the three doshas as well as ones that stimulate, cleanse, or strengthen particular glands or organ systems.

Postures that work on the pelvic area are best for Vata conditions, such as knee/chest pose, locust, plough, cobra, and head and shoulders stand. Headstands are too stimulating for Pitta conditions. Preferred postures for Pitta work on the umbilical area and small intestine such as the bow, shoulder stand, half boat, half wheel, and fish pose. Postures that are best for Kapha focus on the chest, lungs, and abdomen such as back bends, wheel pose, spinal twist, palm tree, and lion pose. Many of these postures improve digestion and absorption, and elimination, thus cleansing and nourishing tissues (including the skin), while toning the body, improving posture, and harmonizing movement.

Sotai

Sotai is a Japanese form of movement and deep breathing that very quickly brings balance to posture, grace to movement, as well as building flexibility and strength. Sotai is easy to learn and manageable for everyone. It is a particularly valuable form of exercise for those who are less strong or experiencing pain. Sotai is taught at macrobiotic centers. Books are available from the Vega Institute in Oroville, California.

Do-In

This is an inductive form of acupressure that has existed since ancient times in the orient. Do-In uses postures, self-massage pounding, tapping, and rubbing to stimulate and rebalance the subtle electromagnetic energies in the body. Do-In is very invigorating and perfect for people of all ages. A short program for morning and/or evening will bring freshness to your living experience.

Taoist Exercise

Involving both mind and body training, these exercises revitalize the organs of the body and strengthen the subtle energies. These exercises are easy to learn but it is best to have a competent, experienced teacher. While most of them do not demand much strength or flexibility, both improve rapidly with these practices. They gently build physical power and confidence while calming and taming the mind.

Tai Chi Chih

A simplified form of Tai Chi formalized by Justin Stone, Tai Chi Chih is soft and gentle in nature and very quick and easy to learn compared to other Tai Chi forms. It swiftly brings peace and a sense of centeredness to the mind and body. Working rather like an active relaxation exercise, it refreshes and invigorates the whole system. This is a wonderful system to use outside surrounded by nature.

Callanetics

Discovered and refined over the last twenty years by Callan Pinckney, Callanetics quickly and safely strengthens, tones, and reshapes your body to give you the beautiful figure nature intended. The exercises activate the body's deepest and largest muscles, the source of a good figure, making them tight, shapely, and beautifully contoured. Callanetics strengthens without impact and is specifically designed to protect the back as well as the joints. Simple and fun to learn, Callanetics delivers fast, visible results. Classes are available nation-wide with certified instructors. Several excellent videos are also available for home practice.

BATHS

Cleansing the surface of our body is considered to be a sacred ritual in parts of India. The body is prepared for bathing by first receiving an oil massage and then during the actual bathing process, prayers are made. To bathe without the initial massage is considered inauspicious.

Although we may not bathe for spiritual reasons, there is much common sense in the Indian bathing described above. Hygiene is an important aspect of daily health care. The more we do for ourselves on a preventative basis, the better.

Take a bath or shower at least once a day. The skin is an organ of excretion and needs to be cleaned regularly to keep fresh and healthy. This is especially true in hot weather when one should bathe, wash, or shower more frequently. A cool bath or quick cold shower can refresh your energy, sharpen your mind, and improve appetite—which tends to diminish in very hot weather. When it is cold and damp out, wash well, but avoid soaking in hot, steamy baths as this will leach the body of minerals and generally weaken the body in times when it needs to be strong and fortified. (In the right circumstances, this can be turned to a person's advantage to cleanse the body of extensive amounts of salts, meat, and dairy.) It is a general rule to only use cool water on your head when washing your hair. Heating the head overstimulates the nervous system and weakens the hair roots.

Cold-bodied Vata people usually like to soak for long periods in hot baths. They are comforted and relaxed by the warmth. To maintain this warm-all-over feeling, either get directly into bed or follow the warm soak with a quick cool shower. This will dilate the pores and peripheral circulation to keep hands and feet warm and sets the skin to glow.

Pitta people feel weakened—even dizzy—by too much heat, including hot baths, steam rooms, and hot tubs. Cool baths and cold showers help keep down their naturally high body heat. This is particularly true in the summer or when sexually over-aroused.

Kapha people like to laze in the bathroom in a luxurious kind of way. They should use warm water and a soft bristle brush or loufa to wash and stimulate their circulation.

Never use soap on the skin. If you feel you cannot give this up, try making your own soap using the following recipe:

½ cup water or herbal tea
1-2 Tbl. almond oil
5 drops essential oil of lemon, orange, mint, basil, juniper, lavender (use one or more in a mix that you like, the total drops totalling 5)
1 cup pure, natural, unperfumed liquid soap
Mix together in the order listed. Use very sparingly and rinse thoroughly.

Always avoid using soap on areas where there are exposed mucous membranes (genitals and anus) and nipples. They need to keep moist to stay balanced and healthy. Even then, the soap you choose should be natural or Ayurvedic. Some people even have allergenic reactions to these. If you have any kind of skin problem, all soaps should be avoided. Soap destroys the natural protective mantle of the skin and removes beneficial bacteria, allowing those that cause odor and infections to proliferate.

Instead of soap, make a paste with flour to lightly scrub and cleanse the skin. It does not change the pH or damage the protective mantle of the skin. If your skin is particularly dry, massage all over with warm sesame oil before you bathe or add oil to the flour paste used for the scrub. Using milk, instead of water, to form the paste will moisten, soften, and nourish the skin. Raw milk is best. It is richer and the fat molecules are larger than those in homogenized milk so they will not congest the skin because they cannot penetrate it.

For Vata constitutions, use chickpea or lentil flour or oatmeal plus oil, milk, or both depending on level of skin dryness.

Pitta constitutions should use barley or rice flours and milk.

Kapha constitutions should use corn or millet flours mixed with a little powdered clay and water.

For inflamed or acned skin, add a pinch of turmeric to your constitutional mixture. Turmeric is a purifying and healing agent.

As you bathe or shower, chant or sing to purify the whole system.

Special Therapeutic Baths

Using essential oils are the most convenient way to make a luxurious bath. However, the initial investment to get top quality oils that really have healing power can be quite steep. If this is not an issue, you will find essential oil combinations for various conditions in the Aromatherapy section.

As an alternative or just for a change, use fresh herbs picked from a garden or found on a country walk. What better end to a long day out in the country than a long bath with fresh herbs full of sweet memories.

Either add fresh herbs directly into the bath tub or use a small cotton or muslin cloth bag full of your herbs of choice that you can suspend in the flow of the hot tap. To this herbal bag, add oatmeal and milk powder to help nourish and soften the skin. When the bath is full use the bag like a soapy wash cloth, rubbing it all over the body to cleanse and stimulate the skin. In the event that you do not have fresh herbs for this, prepare a strong tea from dried herbs, strain, and pour directly into the bath.

Found below are examples of beneficial herbal formulas and the benefits of some individual herbs when you bathe in them.

• Formula for stimulating circulation—pine, larch, juniper, fir

• For relaxation—equal amounts of chamomile, meadow sweet, lime flowers, and a small amount of valerian root

Single Herbs for the Bath . . .

    Angelica—stimulation

    Borage—softens and cleanses

    Chamomile—soothing, relaxing, slightly astringent

    Comfrey—healing and moistening

    Elder—softening, soothing, cleansing

    Fennel—astringent, cleansing, cooling, decreases itching and
      inflammation

Lavender—antiseptic, decreases inflammation
Lovage—deodorant
Marigold—astringent
Mint—refreshing
Rosemary—invigorating, disinfectant
Sage—deodorant
Southernwood—deodorant
Sweet flag—helps with insomnia

Therapeutic Bath Bags

Cleansing Bag—equal amounts dandelion leaves, blackcurrant leaves, scented geranium, and stinging nettles (Dip the nettles in boiling water to neutralize their sting or use gloves when stuffing the bag.)

Invigorating Bag—equal amounts marigold (calendula), pennyroyal or mint, lovage root, and a few pine needles
Cooling and refreshing bag—equal amounts of lemon verbena, rosemary, fennel, and small amount of lemon peel

In Ayurveda there are many excellent bath formulas. Unfortunately, it may be difficult to find some of the individual ingredients. Fortunately, however, Ayurvedic companies in the west are now making bath mixtures available commercially. Refer to the Resource Appendix.

Epsom Salts Baths

This bath is useful to reduce subtle inflammations in the body caused by Pitta aggravating influences such as radiation, increased UV rays, X-rays, and chemical pollutants. The more often you are exposed to these types of influences the more frequently you should take these baths. One every three days, however, is the maximum. Such baths are particularly useful for hospital personnel, computer operators, and those that work around heavy chemicals.

Make a bath deep enough to cover your whole body with fairly hot water. Add four cups of epsom salts. Soak for twenty minutes. Rinse off in cool water or just pat dry and leave the residue on the skin overnight if it does not cause skin irritation.

Epsom salts baths are also helpful in cases of general inflammation, itching, bug bites, and muscle strains.

SUN AND MOON BATHING (Atapa)

Resting in the sun improves the circulation and induces sweating which reduces toxins. So, sunbathing can be cleansing as well as pleasurable. Done in moderation it is both healthy and safe. A half-hour of full sun exposure daily is sufficient. Over-exposure, however, can deeply damage the skin. Always use sunscreen, especially on the face.

People with high Vata dosha usually enjoy the warmth and energy of the sun. When Pitta is high, sun bathing for a short period before noon is best. When Kapha is high, sunbathing for longer periods than either Vata or Pitta (approximately one hour) is usually enough.

Just as resting in the sun warms and stimulates the body, moon bathing calms and cools the system. Traditional texts paint romantic pictures of relaxing on tropical nights on a terrace under a full moon, sipping cool sweet milk from a silver cup while being massaged by gentle cool hands fresh with sandalwood water. For those of us living in colder climates, brief exposure to the moon by an open window is said to reduce high Pitta in both the body and the mind. Full moon is the best time. Be discrete.

TAKING FRESH AIR (Marut)

When I was a child, our old fashioned family doctor would visit the house. The first thing he would do was to fling open the windows and tell my mother to bring me some brown bread and honey.

Fresh air is charged with prana (life force). Whether we are sick or not the body appreciates this precious treat. If you are unable to get into the country to find clean air, a combination air filter and negative ion generator will help give your body a similar charge. Plants in the house also help to clean and charge the air. Indians use holy basil, commonly known as Tulsi, which is said to strongly purify the air while charging the air with negative ions and liberating ozone from the sun's rays.

Be they man-made devices or plants, it is interesting to see how nature has so many solutions if we can discover where to look.

MEDITATION

Meditation can be incorporated into any form of mind training that calms the body and increases the awareness or creates greater focus for any action that is sincere, pure and heartfelt. Benefits of meditation include a greater sense of relaxation in both mind and body, greater flexibility of thinking, an ability to meet situations with freshness and insight, and achieve a greater sense of creativity and joy. From the standpoint of pure physical expression, it can help loosen the knots and tensions trapped in the body by disturbing emotions. It can help to change both facial expression and body posture, thereby softening and strengthening at the same time. These are some of the possible results, but they are not the goals. Attention to the discipline of meditation is what brings results, not desire. Meditation is nectar for the mind as good food is nourishment in the body. Meditation strengthens positive qualities of compassion, patience, and wisdom and frees us of conflicting emotions and erroneous beliefs. It calls for the strongest kind of self-discipline and is an essential ingredient in developing true inner beauty; the deep inner glow that shines stronger as the years go by.

There are many forms of meditation: silent sitting, chanting, praying, walking meditation, meditation that uses visualization or focus on objects, even fighting meditation of the martial arts disciplines. Though often discussed within the context of eastern religions, meditation can be found in almost every tradition in the world if one were to look into their more contemplative practices.

It is best to find a well qualified teacher that you admire and trust. Look at their qualities and the qualities of their students to see if what you observe in them is what you want to develop. If there is a long tradition, examine the result of using their particular discipline over time. Relating to a teacher or at least discussing your experience with like-minded individuals is very helpful. To help you explore the possibilities, there is a list of books and organizations in the Source Appendix.

In terms of which form of meditation is best for each constitution type I feel it is best for each person to follow their natural inclination and grow and deepen from there.

Vata people are naturally attracted to movement and sound. They are highly sensitive, especially to the most subtle forms of energy. Tai Chi, forms of walking meditation and dance are good. Meditation using prayers, song, chants, and musical instruments may also appeal. Tight discipline and long hours of formal, silent, or rigidly still practice can derange Vata mentally.

Pitta people, being very visual, enjoy meditations that use color, images, or beautiful objects. As in all activities they should guard against getting too intense or competitive.

Kapha people find it easy to sit quietly and contemplate. They have a naturally compassionate and devotional nature. To help avoid sleepiness, use incense or perfume in the air to keep the senses alert and take periods of walking outside in between periods of sitting.

For those of you new to the idea of meditation, I have provided some brief instructions for sitting meditation. They are basically from the Tibetan Buddhist tradition, but included are a few other ideas that I have found useful over the years.

Basic Instructions for Sitting Meditation . . .
• Wash your hands, face, and feet.
• Find a quiet, clean, well ordered, well-ventilated space; indoors or outdoors is fine.
• Sit comfortably. If you are in a chair, sit with your back as straight as possible, slightly away from the chair back. Rest your feet together firmly on the ground (barefeet is best). If you prefer, sit cross-legged on the ground upon firm pillows that are high enough to allow your knees to be lower than the level of your navel.
• Tuck your chin in slightly to help relax the back of your neck.

- Rest your tongue behind your front teeth allowing your mouth to be slightly open.
- Draw up the muscles of your lower pelvis.
- Rest your hands on your knees.
- Gently fix your gaze between your knees if you are sitting on a chair or about 18 inches from the point where your legs cross.
- Breathe in through your nose, hold for a moment, then relax the body and allow the breath to go out. Keep your attention on your breath, feeling the sensations in your body as it comes in and goes out. Count 21 breaths like this. If you lose track of the number of breaths you have counted, start again at 1 until you can undistractedly count to 21. After you have done this, just observe the breath as it flows from the tip of your nose and out. If your mind becomes distracted from your breath, just say to yourself the word, "thinking" and resume your attention to the breath.
- Do this for 20 minutes minimum to start with and gradually increase as time and inclination allows.

Try to practice this meditation regularly at about the same time each day. Early morning is best as the body is rested and the world outside is still relatively quiet. It also harmonizes Vata energy in the body which is active at this time.

If you do feel you cannot find enough time in your day for meditation, remember this simple Tibetan saying: "If you have time to breathe then you have time to meditate." Meditation is a state of mind. With a little practice, you will be able to do it anywhere.

Healing Meditation

The following meditation is suitable for addressing physical problems as well as emotional and spiritual difficulties. Practices similar to the one presented here are now used in hospitals and clinics where practitioners recognize the value of meditation and imagery in the healing process. The format presented here is common to many Tibetan practices, but has been placed into a more generic vernacular by Dr. Lobsang Rapgay, a Tibetan Ayurvedic physician and family friend. As I'm sure he would say, "May it benefit many beings."

• Relax the body by tensing then releasing each muscle group. Start with the feet and move to the calves, abdomen, hands, arms, jaws, and facial muscles.

• For a few moments, sit in silent mediation as described earlier.

• Then, for a few minutes, contemplate why you are doing this meditation. Bring to mind the particular problem you need help with and any associated feelings, worries, desires, and so on.

• Think that you are not only asking for yourself to be healed, but for everyone everywhere who suffers.

• Bring to your mind the image of your ideal healer. This may be a particular therapist, a spiritual teacher, God, an enlightened being, or deity. It can even be a geometric form, color, and/or vibration that you associated with healing energy. Take a few moments to bring this image clearly to your minds eye.

• With a sense of respect and invitation, let the healer know that you and other beings are wanting their attention.

• Imagine that the healer is pleased to be asked and agrees to help. This makes you feel happy and you take a moment to feel this good feeling and experience a sense of gratitude.

• Now see white light going out of the ideal healer in all directions to all possible sources of help for your condition. The light returns in rainbow colors, (especially dark blue) to the heart or center of the healer making them even more powerful and full of wisdom and healing energy than before.

• Now the light comes from the heart or center of the healer towards you. As you breathe in, imagine that you are taking in colored light, letting it travel throughout your body, especially to problem areas. (For Vata or Kapha conditions, the light should be mostly dark blue. For Pitta conditions they should be mostly reddish-white.)

• The light dissolves all problems into small dark particles that forms a smokey cloud and leaves your body and passes into the ground as you breathe out.

• Repeat these last two steps 3, 7, or 21 times.
• Once you have received your healing, see this healing energy going to others. Again, breathe in and out to a cycle of 3, 7, or 21 times.
• Have confidence in this process. Feel yourself getting stronger, clearer, more balanced and more self confident than before. As you feel yourself strengthened, the healer image moves to a remote distance, honoring your strength and independence.
• Pause a moment in gratitude for the help the healer has offered you and others. Then let the image of the healer completely dissolve into space.

If formal meditation does not appeal to you and you cannot take the time for a full skilled relaxation session, try the following simple yogic technique. Like so many simple things, with a little practice and regularity in its use, this exercise can become very powerful and transformative. And, it only takes a few moments and can be done anywhere. It is an excellent natural tranquilizer.
• Sit quietly and comfortably with your back straight, yet relaxed, and your chin a little tucked in.
• Rest the tip of your tongue behind your front teeth throughout this exercise.
• Exhale completely and loudly though your mouth
• Close your mouth and inhale quietly through your nose to a silent count of 4.
• Hold the breath for 7 counts.
• Exhale as before to a count of 8.

The exact speed is not important, but the ratio of 4:7:8 is. Repeat the whole process 3 more times, making a total of 4 cycles.

SLEEP
In India, sleep is called the "wet nurse of the world" because it is nurturing, nourishing, and regenerating. There are two types of sleep: deep dreamless sleep that restores the physical body and active dreaming sleep, called REM (Rapid Eye Movement) sleep, that helps clear

the mind of conflicting emotions.

Sleep is a great healer and strengthener. Along with other positive lifestyle practices, adequate sleep helps to enhance a fresh, clean, vital and beautiful mind and body. It has many of the same elements as skilled relaxation and some of the side benefits of meditation which is why it is said that when one cannot get enough sleep, these practices will help one become recharged and refreshed.

The hours of darkness are the healthiest times to sleep. Sleeping during the day is not advised as it is said to produce toxins or ama in both the body and the mind. There are some exceptions though, such as for the very young or the elderly, and for persons that are weak from illness, tired from too much sex or intoxication, overwork, or emotional distress. A 10 to 20 minute cat nap can actually be helpful to recharge a busy Vata type person if it is taken in the early afternoon. Longer naps are also sometimes advised in very hot weather between noon and three or four o'clock in the afternoon—in some cultures called "siesta" time.

Like so many things, Ayurveda considers sleep needs to be individual. Vata people tend to have light, restless sleep that is variable in quality for short periods of time (4-6 hours nightly). As they love excitement and can easily over extend themselves, Vatas may need to take time for naps, relaxation, and meditation to supplement sleep. High Vata energy people must learn to nurture themselves with quality rest as they are most susceptible to the disturbing influences of modern city life, noise, pollution, overcrowding and emotional stress. An early night after a warm oil massage and a fragrant warm bath is an excellent way to relax and recharge to keep good looking despite a busy and rather chaotic lifestyle.

Pitta people usually sleep easily, lightly, and wake alert. They usually do best with 6 to 8 hours of sleep, but of all the constitutional types they can survive getting very little sleep several nights in a row. Their hard driving nature and concern for achievement can interfere with both the quality and quantity of sleep. Anxiety and worldly worries are the main causes for their insomnia. Pitta people need to pace their activity and give themselves time for their achievements. Taking a cool shower, sipping a sweet drink, and meditating in the moonlight help to unwind high Pitta energy.

Kapha people love to rest and take life as it comes. They rarely have difficulty sleeping and enjoy long deep sleep which lasts often longer than eight hours. Yet they awake refreshed. Kapha types need to watch that they don't sleep too much, however, as sleep is by its own nature Kapha producing and can lead to weight gain and mental heaviness. Early to bed and early to rise will help Kapha types be healthy, wealthy, and wise! Interestingly, this rhyme was invented for children who, by virtue of their stage in life, are more Kapha.

Please note that as we get older the Vata qualities in our being naturally increase which is one good reason why older people need less sleep at night and can get by on cat naps. This is a normal pattern and special treatment is only needed when there is long term exhaustion. Ayurveda teaches us to listen to the body's demand to rest if one is tired. If, however, you have difficulty feeling refreshed by sleep, follow the suggestions below . . .

General Advice for Peaceful Sleep

• Wash your hands, face, and feet and clean your mouth and teeth before sleeping.

• Do not eat or drink for two hours before bedtime, especially very spicy or greasy foods, or caffienated soft drinks, black tea, or coffee. Caffeine not only keeps you awake, but makes sleep more restless. Also, avoid alcoholic beverages before bedtime. Although they may initially help one to get to sleep, it often makes one rouse in the early hours and reduces the quality of rest the remainder of the night.

• Meditate briefly to clear the cares of the day before you close your eyes.

• Sleep in a quiet, slightly cool, well ventilated space away from smoke or the smell of food. These smells keep your nervous system on alert at a time when it should be totally relaxed.

• Lay on your right side to promote the most restful sleep. Breathing mostly through your left nostril naturally calms and cools the body. You may even close your right nostril to help with this.

• Sleep with your head in the east for the most meditative sleep and pleasant dreams. Sleeping with your head in the west evokes disturbing dreams and restless sleep. Sleeping with your head in the south works with the polarity of the earth to charge and heal the body. Your head in the north can be draining of energy. If you are ill, never sleep this way as it is considered to make recovery much slower and more difficult.

• To feel more naturally relaxed and secure, try to sleep facing the main bedroom door and next to a wall. A sleeping companion, human or animal, is also helpful for nervous Vata people.

Useful Suggestions For Insomnia and Improving the Quality of Your Sleep

Try any one or combination of these suggestions for improving the quality of your sleep . . .

• Exercise during the day helps cleanse the body of adrenalin that builds up due to stress and keeps the body tense and mind overactive.

• Practice skilled relaxation during the day or when you get home from work. You can also do this just before retiring. Relaxation exercises condition you to develop increases of alpha brainwave stimulation. Do such exercises in a place not associated with sleep, but relaxation; i.e. not your bed, but perhaps a lounge chair, couch, or floor. Doing such an exercise before bed can settle you down so that you do not go to bed in a overly tired or mentally overactive state.

• Exercise before bed by gently stretching the spine, neck, and shoulder areas where the most tension accumulates in the day. One technique is to lie on the floor on your back and draw up your knees and clutch them. Rock back and forth on your spine to loosen the spine and increase even flow of circulation throughout the spine. This helps the whole body to relax.

• Take a luke-warm bath. Pat yourself dry and get directly into bed. Hot showers and baths stimulate circulation, increasing the heart rate, making it harder to settle down to rest.

• Herbal decoctions added to the bath help slow both the body and mind into a quieter, more peaceful mode of being.

Herbal Bath for Sound Sleep

Bring one gallon of water to the boil. Add the following herbs:

    1½ cups chamomile
    1 cup meadow sweet
    1 cup lime flowers
    ½ cup valerian root

Steep these herbs for 30 minutes, strain, and add to a deep bath. Add a few tablespoons of sesame oil to the bath as well (This can be done, even if one does not make the herbal mixture.) This finely coats the skin as you bathe, reducing Vata qualities of tension and restlessness.

• Wear natural fiber night clothes and try to use a bed and bed coverings that are also natural: a cotton futon, cotton or silk linens, and thick cotton or wool blankets, or a down comforter. Natural fibers do not interfere with the natural flow of electromagnetic energy in the body as do man-made fibers. (If you use an electric blanket to warm your bed, turn it off and unplug it before you go to sleep——for the same reasons.) Use natural, unscented washing powders for bed clothes to avoid allergies that can cause skin reactions and headaches.

• Massage the scalp and bottoms of the feet with warm sesame or brahmi oil. Use a towel on your pillow and put sport socks on your feet to avoid staining the bed sheets and covers.

• Use essential oils in a warm bath, in a diffuser, on a light bulb ring, or sprinkled on a handkerchief and pinned to your pillow. Try combinations like 1) chamomile, lavender, cypress, marjoram, good if there is also some digestive upset, and 2) sandalwood or clary sage plus melissa, orange blossom, rose, ylang ylang or juniper, good if the body is overheated.

• Use a negative ion generator. Negative ions ease the mind, please the senses and relax the body. Negative ions are naturally in high concentration near the ocean, waterfalls, and in forests—places associated with relaxation and pleasure. Sleep near a Tulsi (Holy Basil) plant if you can find one. Such practices help to counteract positive ions often found in urban environments.

• Listen to quiet, calming music.

• Drink a cup of warm spiced milk in the late evening. Raw cows milk is best for Vata types so long as they are not lactose intolerant. Soy or goat milk is better for Pitta and Kapha types. *The Ayurvedic Cookbook,* by Amadea Morningstar has a number of interesting recipes for such drinks with guidelines as to the appropriateness for the different constitutional types. Here are a few samples:

> 1 cup raw milk
> ½ teaspoon freshly ground nutmeg

Bring milk to a boil, reduce heat and stir in the nutmeg. Simmer for five minutes, strain and serve. Add one tablespoon of old brandy for extra warming as needed. If used regularly, Kapha types should add a little dry ginger and use goat milk. Pitta types should drink this drink lukewarm with a small amount of raw sugar or maple syrup.

> 1 cup of soy milk
> dash of cinnamon
> ½ teaspoon of sweetener (honey for Vata and Kapha types, and maple syrup, rice or barley malt for Pitta types).

This is a good drink if you are hungry at bedtime, but do not want to eat.

• Drink herbal teas that have a natural sedative effect. There are several commercial blends available, but you can also make your own. Use one teaspoon of herb per cup of boiling water, allowing the herbs to steep for at least ten minutes before straining. When using seeds, crush them slightly first to hasten their brewing process.

Sedative herbs include: bergamot, chamomile, elderflower, lemon verbena, passion flower, vervain, violet leaves and flowers, poppy seed, skullcap, valerian (jatamamsi), bhringaraj, seeds of anise, fennel, and dill.

If there is indigestion associated with insomnia, use peppermint, mullein, nutmeg. In this case use with milk rather than water.

Try this particular formula for insomnia:

1 teaspoon lemon balm
1 teaspoon marjoram
1 teaspoon hops
1 teaspoon crushed anise

Make an infusion of this mixture in 1 pint of boiling water. Take one cup before bedtime.

• Never read, watch T.V., listen to music, write, even think in bed. Allow your bed to only be associated with restful, relaxing sleep.

• To reduce anxiety about going to sleep, develop a routine that works and stick to it. The body loves routine and will learn useful behaviors more quickly if they are done regularly, like a positive ritual.

AROMAS, COLORS, SOUNDS, GEMS

"Matter is energy and what seems solid is but a static appearance of innumerable subtle moving forces."
David Frawley

Ayurveda teaches that the world and everything we experience is no more than the play of energy that condenses from primordial space; energy in different forms but behaving with cosmic intelligence, according to the laws of nature. We have already discussed how the human body is viewed as being formed by the cohesion of the five elements of ether, air, fire, water, and earth which combine to form Vata (ether and air), Pitta (fire and water), and Kapha (water and earth) doshas and these doshas give the body various distinctive characteristics. These elements and the intelligence or rules by which they come together are types of energy. Looking to western tradition, it is energy which has been recognized by quantum physicists as the true building block of the universe, both inside of us and everywhere else.

Ayurveda teaches that on the most basic level human beings are energy bodies dancing in the energy soup of our whole universe — not distinct from it but deeply, fundamentally connected to it. Realizing this, it is easy to understand why the world around us influences our whole being down to smaller than atomic level. Not only does our world influence us, but it does so according to cosmic rules. The rule that "like increases like" is demonstrated in how energies outside of the body that are like the ones inside of the body will increase those like energies in the body. And as has been described at some length, opposite qualities to those inside the body help to balance the energies in the body.

99

How these outside energies influence our body is through the various sense fields that we have, each of which is associated with a particular dosha of the body. The senses themselves, having various qualities, demonstrate their affinity to particular doshas.

Vata, a combination of ether and air elements, has an affinity to that which produces resonance (sound) and sense of presence (touch).

Pitta, a combination of fire and water elements, has an affinity to that which is exposed by the light of fire (sight) and our awareness that something is present in space and being able to discern what it is. Thus Pitta helps us to be aware of sights, colors, and forms.

Kapha, a combination of earth and water elements, has an affinity to deeper senses of appreciation for distinction through smell and taste; taste which not only is associated with the tongue, but has an actual quality of savoring and satisfaction.

People who have a dominantly Vata constitution will thus be most strongly influenced by sound and touch, Pitta constitutions by sights, and Kapha constitutions by tastes and smells.

As each individual is a unique mixture of Vata, Pitta, and Kapha energy, each will have a proportionately varying ability to "sense" the world around them. This inherent sensitivity to specific forms of sensory impression based on constitutional type is the basis for the use of the subtle therapies that utilize aroma, color, gems, fabrics, sound and prayers.

The *Vedas* were written in ancient times when life was not necessarily more harmonious, but certainly more natural. People were in closer contact with the earth and the changes of the seasons. Their experience of the natural world was fuller. Today we have traded this type of direct and rich experience for comfort and convenience. More people now live in cities, spending more of their waking hours in man-made environments. Simple things like light and heat that once ruled our work and sleep patterns have become controllable at the flick of a switch. Foods from all over the world are available to us year round, abolishing seasonal selection. Seemingly, we have more control, but the further we get from natural rhythms, the more stressed our daily living becomes. Why? Because on a fundamental level so many modern conveniences disturb the natural flow of our body energy. Given that we cannot all drop out and get back to nature, what can be done to help restore our own natural balance in modern times?

Lifestyle and diet have been discussed. I now want to more closely examine the more subtle therapies alluded to earlier. I do so not only for a sense of completeness and because there is increasing interest in them, but also because of their direct and strong influence on the doshas, which in turn influence our sense of well being.

Ayurveda is not a dogma, but a growing body of information aimed at helping people towards a full and rich life. So, while much of the information in this chapter is traditional, I have also integrated some modern research data and applications that are in keeping with the spirit and philosophy of Ayurveda.

A BRIEF HISTORY OF AROMATHERAPY, EAST AND WEST

Aromatherapy as we know it today is the revival of a branch of herbal medicine that has been honored and treasured for centuries by peoples throughout the world. Along with precious metals, gems, fabrics, and spices, naturally fragrant oils were highly prized throughout the ancient world. Popular in Egyptian times, the Phoenicians exported oils to the Arabs, Greeks, and Romans. Hippocrates, known as the "father of medicine," prescribed fumigations and fomentations using these precious oils for their medicinal properties. The Romans favored them for perfume, to adorn their bodies, hair, clothing, even linens.

With the fall of the Roman Empire, knowledge of aromatics travelled to and flourished in Persian and Arab countries. Avicenna (980-1037 AD), a gifted Arabian physician, scholar, and profuse writer, devoted an entire book to the rose—the most cherished flower in Islamic tradition.

The Crusades brought natural oils back to Europe. By the late 15th century native European herbs such as lavender, sage, and rosemary were being distilled. These aromatic preparations were very popular during the Renaissance period when they were considered to be the best protection against epidemics. At the end of the 17th century, the use of aromatics became divided into perfumery and alchemy. Essential oils continued to be used for their medicinal properties until around 1818 when the French published a code of medicines and pharmacopeia which strongly discredited the healing aspects of aromas and essential oils. They continued to be used in perfumes, cosmetics, and foodstuffs, however.

In 1928, a French chemist named Gattefosse led the revival of this art. Dr. Jean Valnet, another Frenchman, published "Aromatherapie" in 1964, again establishing aromatics as a bonified herbal treatment. One of his students, Madame Marguerite Maury, was the first to again use essential oils for their perfume and medicinal properties in cosmetics. Her long-term aim was to create strictly personal aromatic complexes adapted to an individual's temperament and particular health problems—a truly Ayurvedic perspective, viewing the body, mind, and spirit as a totality for treatment and care. Essential oils are now widely used by the natural cosmetic industry and are gradually re-gaining acceptance in the field of medicine.

In India there is evidence that distilled floral waters were used 5000 years ago. Crude distillation apparatae was recently discovered in Pakistan which has been linked to the Indus Valley civilization. Archaeologists have found perfume containers dated from 3000 BC, confirming that people were using aromatic herbal preparations then. Vedic literature from 2000 BC lists over 700 substances, including cinnamon, ginger, myrrh, and sandalwood and describes their uses for body and mind, suggesting that this was a developed art of healing. Referred to as "attars," which means not only perfume, but smoke, wind, odor, or essence, they were used widely in religious ceremony to help quiet the mind and deepen meditation. They remain a part of Ayurvedic medicine which has perfected the art of incense making and body oil preparation. Medicinally they are considered most helpful when the primary cause of illness is a mental/emotional disturbance. They are recommended especially in conditions of stress and depression. Their effectiveness for skin disorders and natural influence on the emotions makes them one of the best vehicles for Ayurvedic cosmetics.

WHAT ARE ESSENTIAL OILS?

"*Oshadi*" is the Indian word used for healing plants. Literally, it means "giver of life" or "carrier of light." This word perfectly describes the action of pure essential oils.

Formed in plant cells by the action of the sun, essential oils are reservoirs of solar healing power. They are the source of all fragrance in flowers, leafs, spices, fruits, and aromatic woods, and herbs. Described as the "life blood" of the plant, Marcel Lavabre, a French aromatherapist went one step further when he said "essential oils are the ultimate manifestation of a plant's *joie de vivre*, or enjoyment of life." Such aromas are invigorating both to body and mind, please the sense, and bring us in touch with nature wherever we encounter them.

Many essential oils are antiseptic and antibacterial. Some are proving helpful for viral infections by boosting immune function. Others have the potential to stimulate healthy cell renewal and growth. Useful not only to bring health and delicious fragrance to the body, they also have been shown to regulate and restore balance to mental functioning. The healing power of medicinal quality essential oils is, therefore, extensive and profound. Thankfully, today, they are being restored to their rightful place in the pharmacopeia of herbal medicine. In Europe they are rapidly gaining acceptance in conventional medical circles. For example, lavender essential oil is used for severe burns while essential oil of rose is used to treat addictions, depression, and other mental health conditions where a mild tranquilizer is recommended.

Each oil or oil combination has a distinct profile or personality that makes it useful not only for particular conditions, but also personality types. This makes it interesting from the point of view of Ayurveda as a particular oil can be suitable to relieve a specific condition as well as the underlying mental state that contributed to the manifestation of a given symptom. For example, clary sage is used both to calm inflamed skin and alleviate mental irritability, anxiety, tension, and fatigue. Thus, this is an excellent oil for a case where increased Pitta due to work pressure has led to the manifestation of a skin rash. Thus clary sage has helped on two levels to balance the Pitta dosha.

PATHWAYS AND INFLUENCES OF ESSENTIAL OILS

Essential oils are believed to influence the body and mind through two principle pathways, through the skin and via the sense of smell.

When essential oils are applied to the skin in body oil, perfume oil, lotion, spray mist, or placed in bath water, they easily permeate the skin because their molecular structure is so small. Entering most readily through the hair follicles, pores, and interstitial fluid that is around all skin cells, they reach the fine capillaries of the blood and lymph system. Thus they are carried throughout the entire body to all cells, crossing even the blood-brain barrier to act on the outer portions of the brain.

When one smells a fragrance, it is the tiny droplets of airborn essential oils which have triggered a response in the olfactory epithelium or smell sensor in the roof of the nose. From there it is just one nerve synapse to the limbic system of the brain which regulates motor activities, primary drives, emotions, and memories. Impulses are then transmitted to the hypothalamus which regulates such bodily functions as temperature, thirst, hunger, blood sugar level, growth, sleep and wake patterns, sexual arousal, and the emotions. From there the pituitary is stimulated next, which activates the endocrine system which in turn controls digestion, emotional and sexual behaviour, responses to stress, and all metabolic processes.

My personal sense is that there is another level beyond the dramatic influences on the body and mind; a level on which these life essences of plants are able to rally the life force in human beings, becoming an energy and inspiration to seek well being—a spiritual level if you wish.

Essential oils take as little as fifteen minutes to influence the entire body, mind, and spirit. Their effect is not cumulative as all traces of their physical presence in the body leaves after two to three hours.

QUALITY OF ESSENTIAL OILS

With the growing popularity of aromatherapy, more and more product lines are appearing. Most claim natural, even organic origin. Many, however, are perfume rather than medicinal quality and are stretched by being carried in vegetable oils or alcohol. These inferior types may smell nice, but do not have the beneficial qualities one is looking for. If one is wanting the highest grades with the most beneficial effects, some of the companies listed in the Source Appendix at the end of this volume will be helpful.

Otherwise, please note:

1) Good quality oils are sold in amber colored bottles with dropper tops.

2) They should not feel oily when rubbed between the fingers.

3) They should not leave a greasy spot on a blotter or tissue after evaporation.

4) They should not break up or leave a milky trace in water.

5) They should not smell of alcohol

6) They should have been stored at room temperature or cooler and out of direct sunlight.

SELECTION OF ESSENTIAL OILS FOR EACH DOSHA

In Ayurveda, aromas are selected to balance the doshas by their qualities. This will include their smell; whether they have a heating or cooling effect on the body; and the particular emotions they help to balance in the mind.

Oils for Vata should be sweet or slightly sour, warming, nourishing, lubricating, and calming to the nervous system and mind in general. As always the rule with Vata is moderation, thus especially because essential oils are so powerful, they should only be used in the concentration and proportions as given in the recipes. In the case of Vata, very strong smell will have an aggravating effect. Useful fragrances for balancing Vata include:

clary sage	geranium	cinnamon
cypress	clove	jasmine
musk	orange	rose
sandalwood (when applied warm)		

The best base or carrier oils for Vata is cold pressed sesame oil. It is warming, grounding, nourishing, and deeply calming and lubricating. It is the only oil known to be able to penetrate all seven layers of the skin. Avocado, carrot seed, and Vitamin E oils are useful to bring extra nourishment to extra dry skin.

Oils for Pitta should be sweet or slightly astringent or bitter; cooling to the body; and balancing for such emotions as agitation, impatience, anger, and aggression. Suitable Pitta-balancing fragrances are:

chamomile	gardenia	jasmine
honeysuckle	lotus	lemon grass
melissa	mint	rose
rosewood	sandalwood	vertivert

Traditionally, rose and sandalwood are used extensively in Ayurvedic cosmetics. Sandalwood is used on the third eye region (the middle of the forehead) to calm the mind and cool the head for prayer and meditation.

The best carrier oil for Pitta is coconut. This is a little thick for western tastes. Sunflower, safflower, jojoba oils and even sesame oil, providing it is mixed with cooling essential oils, are excellent substitutes. Ghee, clarified butter, that has been "washed" with water in a silver or copper vessel is highly prized in India for its healing and Pitta reducing qualities. It, too, is pretty thick and greasy. Unless you live in an unusually dry climate, it is best used only medicinally. One-hundred-year-old ghee which has been "washed" more than 100 times is considered a panacea.

Essential oils for Kapha should be pungent, slightly astringent or bitter, spicy, light, woody, warming yet stimulating to the mind and body. Such fragrances include:

cedar	cinnamon	musk
eucalyptus	myrrh	patchouli
pine	sage	

Eucalyptus is used primarily in a diffuser to help clear the head and purify the air. It can also be rubbed on the chest to relieve congestion or dabbed on herpes blisters (or other forms of blisters) in a strong dilution. However, it is generally applied directly to the skin only once highly diluted and even then, its over-powering aroma is considered too strong for general cosmetic purposes.

Carrier oils for Kapha include mustard, flax seed, jojoba, olive, and almond oils.

All carrier oils that are from vegetable sources should be cold pressed and organic if possible. Cold pressed oils are rich in Vitamin B and E and contain their own natural preservatives. Organic quality is always best as it is richer and more vital. It is also free of pesticides and chemical fertilizers that become concentrated in the extraction process. These chemicals are apt to collect in the skin and lead to premature aging.

WAYS TO USE ESSENTIAL OILS

What follows are descriptions of the methods by which essential oils are applied or absorbed into the body.

Diffuser—a small piece of equipment that consists of an electric air pump, oil chamber, and glass nebulizer that disperses microparticles of essential oils into the air. These particles are so small that they remain suspended in the air to purify, pleasantly perfume, and transform the atmosphere of an entire room, thus effecting those who come into that space. As they make noise and are relatively powerful in getting the scent into the room, such diffusers are used for short periods of time only.

Ceramic Diffuser—powered by a candle which heats a solution of water and essential oils in a vessel that sits above the candle heat source. Gentle and quiet, it is especially useful when a quiet, restful atmosphere is needed. These are suitable during massages, for study, meditation, and at bedtime.

Aromatic Potteries—small clay bottles that hold enough oil to perfume a car, linen chest, or closet.

Light Bulb Rings—made of cardboard or ceramic material that has been saturated with an essential oil. When the light bulb that they surround or are close to is turned on, the heat causes the aroma to be diffused into the room.

Incense—one of the oldest ways of utilizing essential oils. Herbs are dried and used separately or in combination to create various atmospheric and therapeutic effects. In Native American ritual, individual herbs like sage or sweet grass are pressed into sticks, blocks or tight bundles. Oriental tradition is to finely powder the desired aromatic substances to form joss sticks, incense cones, or powders that are burned on charcoal. Traditional incense is used for prayer and meditation, but is useful anytime to bring a calm, clear atmosphere to a room. There are also specific medicinal incenses, noted especially in Tibetan Ayurvedic sources.

Cosmetics—oils, lotions, shampoos, conditioners, steams, masks, compressed bath salts, shower gels, etc.. Essential oils have the unique ability to penetrate through all the layers of the skin, thus are very effective to moisturize, heal and regenerate the skin. The Source Appendix will give you suppliers of cosmetics that have quality essential oils. Otherwise, high quality essential oils are easily mixed into all kinds of natural cosmetics such as oils, lotions, and soaps to enhance their effects.

BATH OIL COMBINATIONS

Usually essential oils are used in combinations called "synergies." Synergies are blended to mutually enhance the aromas, medicinal properties, and amplify the healing energy of all the oils used. A good synergy will naturally appeal to the individual's nose and the mind and thus be appropriate to the constitution, temperament, symptom, cause, and circumstance of the individual.

Mixing synergies is a fine art. The selection of bath combinations found below will give you some idea of their potential. Recipes for massage oil synergies, other products and conditions they are used for are found in the skin care and treatment chapter.

Bath Oil Synergies—To a warm bath, into which you will immerse yourself, add the following combinations for the therapeutics effects indicated . . .

Cleansing—
4 drops basil
3 drops rosemary
3 drops lemon

Normal Skin—
5 drops neroli
3 drops rose
1 cup milk
1 Tbl. honey

Oily Skin—
5 drops basil
2 drops lemon
2 cups cider vinegar

Dry Skin—
6 drops rosa mosquita
6 drops bergamot
2 Tbl. sesame oil
1 Tbl. honey

Tired Blemished Skin—
6 drops clary sage
2 drops lemon
2 cups cider vinegar

Blemished Skin—
5 drops tea tree oil
5 drops lavender
2 cups cider vinegar

TABLE 2. AROMA THERAPY CHART

	NORMAL	DRY	OILY	MATURE	ACNE	INFLAMMED	ECZEMA	SENSITIVE	ITCHY	CHAPPED	WRINKLES	BLEMISHES/SCARS	CONGESTED	TIRED/FLABBY	CELLULITE	VARICOSE/THREAD VEINS	INCREASES PHOTOSENSITIVITY OR IRRITATING
BERGAMOT	✓	✓	✓	✓		✓	✓					✓					✓
CEDAR			✓		✓		✓		✓				✓				✓
CHAMOMILE		✓			✓	✓	✓	✓	✓							✓	
CLARY SAGE	✓					✓								✓			
CYPRESS			✓				✓						✓	✓	✓	✓	
EUCALYPTUS						✓											✓
FENNEL		✓	✓	✓							✓			✓	✓		
FRANKINCENSE		✓		✓						✓	✓						
GERANIUM	✓	✓	✓	✓	✓	✓	✓						✓	✓	✓	✓	
JASMINE	✓	✓	✓	✓		✓		✓	✓					✓			
JUNIPER			✓	✓	✓	✓	✓						✓	✓	✓	✓	
LAVENDER	✓		✓	✓	✓	✓	✓					✓			✓		✓
LEMON			✓	✓	✓	✓			✓		✓		✓	✓		✓	
MELISSA				✓									✓	✓	✓		
MYRRH	✓	✓		✓		✓	✓		✓		✓						
NEROLI	✓	✓	✓	✓		✓						✓				✓	✓
ORANGE			✓					✓						✓			
PATCHOULI	✓			✓	✓	✓	✓			✓				✓	✓		✓
PEPPERMINT	✓			✓	✓	✓			✓				✓	✓	✓	✓	
ROSE	✓	✓		✓	✓	✓		✓								✓	
ROSEMARY		✓	✓	✓	✓		✓								✓	✓	
ROSEWOOD	✓	✓		✓	✓	✓								✓			
SANDALWOOD	✓	✓	✓	✓	✓	✓	✓		✓	✓						✓	
TEA TREE			✓		✓	✓							✓				
YLANG YLANG	✓	✓	✓														

TABLE 2. AROMA THERAPY CHART (Cont.)

	ANTISEPTIC	ASTRINGENT	ANTIBIOTIC	DEODORANT	REFRESHING	UPLIFTING	MENTAL FATIGUE	RELAXING	NERVOUS TENSION	HYSTERIA	RESTLESSNESS	ANGER	INSOMNIA	FEAR/ANXIETY	HAIR LOSS	DANDRUFF	NAIL CARE
BERGAMOT			✓	✓	✓	✓		✓			✓			✓			
CEDAR	✓							✓	✓	✓				✓	✓	✓	
CHAMOMILE	✓						✓	✓	✓	✓	✓	✓	✓	✓			
CLARY SAGE		✓		✓	✓	✓	✓		✓	✓			✓				
CYPRESS		✓		✓								✓		✓			
EUCALYPTUS	✓	✓	✓	✓	✓		✓		✓								
FENNEL	✓																
FRANKINCENSE	✓	✓						✓	✓	✓	✓		✓	✓			
GERANIUM	✓	✓		✓		✓			✓					✓		✓	
JASMINE	✓				✓	✓			✓					✓			
JUNIPER	✓	✓	✓		✓		✓		✓		✓		✓	✓		✓	
LAVENDER	✓		✓	✓	✓	✓		✓	✓				✓	✓	✓	✓	
LEMON	✓	✓	✓				✓									✓	✓
MELISSA					✓						✓	✓	✓	✓			
MYRRH	✓	✓						✓					✓				
NEROLI			✓				✓		✓	✓	✓		✓	✓			
ORANGE		✓							✓								
PATCHOULI	✓					✓	✓	✓				✓					
PEPPERMINT	✓	✓		✓	✓		✓		✓								
ROSE	✓	✓		✓	✓	✓			✓				✓	✓			
ROSEMARY		✓					✓	✓	✓						✓	✓	
ROSEWOOD	✓			✓		✓		✓	✓								
SANDALWOOD		✓				✓		✓	✓	✓			✓	✓		✓	
TEA TREE	✓		✓	✓													
YLANG YLANG		✓				✓			✓	✓		✓	✓	✓	✓		

General Detox—
3 drops geranium
3 drops rosemary
3 drops juniper
2 drops lavender

Revitalizer—
2 drops fennel
4 drops juniper
2 drops rosemary

Sunburn—
6 drops peppermint
9 drops lavender
3 Tbl. jojoba
1 Tbl. honey

Nervous Exhaustion—
2 drops basil
4 drops geranium
4 drops lavender

Pick-Me Up—
3 drops clary sage
3 drops bergamot
3 drops ylang

For more information about the essential oils suitable for particular skin types, skin complaints, and states of mind, check the Aroma Therapy Chart provided (pps. 110-111).

COLOR THERAPY

Ayurveda has always acknowledged the healing power of color. Color is another type of energy vibration received primarily through the eyes, but also—although not to as great an extent—through the skin. Colors have affinity to different body tissues and the potential to either balance or disrupt the three doshas. This is quickly evident by observing the states of mind that different colors can elicit. Take just a moment to reflect on the emotions that surface as you visualize green, red, blue, and yellow. Reactions to colors may vary to some extent among individuals due to conditioning, culture, etc., but you will more than likely find many people have similar experiences as yourself.

Color can be used to further beauty and balance by being selective in your choice of them for home decor, clothing, even the color of your car. Drinking water from colored bottles that have stood in the sun for several hours is a traditional way of "taking color" into the body. The water becomes infused with the color's vibrations and is thus taken directly into the tissues. The same method can be used for oils and all other liquid cosmetics. Theo Gimbel, a color therapist from Switzerland, has developed colored light therapy using banks of electric lights placed on walls in a room in specific patterns to elicit therapeutic responses. Modern technology-based therapies such as Dr. John Downing's Lumatron are intended to have both physiological and psychological benefits, based on an understanding of the workings of our central and autonomic nervous systems and brain chemistry.

Whatever impacts our physiology and psychology is always reflected in our physical appearance and expression. Thus, as color will have an effect on our internal organs as well as our moods, facial contours, lines, skin tone and expression are in part indicators of whatever impact colors have on us. Just in terms of their impact on our expression, colors that are uplifting to us will create a countenance that reflects kindness and generosity. Such expression is infinitely more alluring than one darkened by fear and jealousy. A body carried with confidence is more appealing than one twisted by worry. Surrounding ourselves with uplifting colors and an environment that generally creates positive visual impressions can have a strong impact on how we present ourselves and interact with our world.

Colors for Vata

The rule with Vata is always moderation. Red, orange, yellow, or white are useful because they are warming, energizing, and mind clearing. At the same time, they may be too intense. Pastels and muted shades of these warm colors are best. Greens and blues can be worn to calm the more intense, warmer colors. Avoid black, brown, and grays.

Colors for Pitta

White, blue, and green are balancing to Pitta dosha. Black and very intense colors of any shade should be avoided.

Colors for Kapha

Kapha needs rich and warming colors. Red, purple, gold, and yellow are best. White and pale shades of blue, green, or pink are too sedating for them. Black, grays, or brown are fine in moderation.

COLOR	AFFECTED DOSHA	PSYCHO-PHYSICAL IMPACT	EXCESS CAUSES . . .
Red	Useful for V & K. Aggravates P	enrichers & heats blood, pinks cheeks, helps circulation, vitality, strength Psych . . .stimulating, exciting, activating	inflammations, cravings, aggression
Orange	Useful for V&K Aggravates P in excess	warming & healing, increases sexual energy, clears congestion, brings luster to skin Psych . . .joy, lightness, release, pleasure	renunciation of the world
Yellow	Useful for V&K May aggrav. P	aids digestion, promotes longevity Psych . . .intelligence & detachment	loss of reason, direction, & irritability
Green	Useful for K&V Increases P in excess	calms hyperactivity promotes physical balance Psych . . . tranquility, refreshes, improves judgement	increases bile indecision, jealousy, frustration
Blue	Useful for P Increases V&K in excess	calms, cools, heals recharges Psyche . . . relaxes, unwinds	congestion, stupefaction excessive intro-spection

| Violet | Useful to P&K Increases V | calms, lightens, sharpens senses Psych . . .inner balance, peacefulness, dignity, compassion | Heightened sensuality, disturbing the senses |

About White . . .when used appropriately, white has a purifying quality. However, if used in excess (like wearing all white continually) may cause an increase in pride.

About Black . . .if used in excess can attract negativity and increase rage and hatred.

SOUND

In past times when people were living and working together in smaller communities they would sing together. Singing strengthened their bond and contributed to the more aesthetic achievements in their work. Today this is rare and the "noise" in our life is more prevalent than the harmonies of nature of the past. Traffic, machines, electrical appliances, radios, and T.V. are a major part of daily experience. Modern "noise" or unwanted sound is so pervasive that unless we take a break to the wilderness or experience total power outage and closed roads, we accept it as normal and become unconscious of the impact it has on us.

Sound, like everything else our minds and bodies perceive, can either balance or unbalance the doshas. The *Rishis*, the original authors of Ayurvedic texts, did not have to cope with the same level of auditory abuse as we do today. They were, however, well aware of how noises and unharmonious sounds imbalance and how particular sounds rebalance. For example, singing together tends to remove feelings of estrangement, tenseness, and fear. However, some forms of music have been shown to be disruptive to life force. It has been observed that rap music kills plant life. Gangs are known to listen to rap which may be a contributing factor to their lack of appreciation for order and tendencies towards group violence.

Singing, chanting, playing an instrument or even listening to music helps to restore harmony to our whole living space. Positive sound can transform any place or space into a sanctuary of peace and true pleasure. Many Indian instruments, for example, were designed originally to benefit the body and mind of the listener, and various pieces of music, called ragas, were written to purposefully bring harmony throughout the day, aiding waking, working, digestion, relaxing, sleeping, etc.

Chanting mantras, single or groups of specific syllables, though often associated with spiritual discipline, are also used in Ayurveda for their balancing, nurturing, and rejuvenating effect. Here are a few mantras, or sacred sounds that relate more closely to beauty . . .

OM—empowers the spirit, clears the mind, and increases Ojas—that which creates the glow in health and beauty.

SHREEM—increases the power of feminine energy for health and beauty.

RAM—activates protective energy.

HUM—strengthens all bodily functions.

AYM—attracts the wisdom goddess, Sarasvati.

KREEM—empowers home-made cosmetics.

KLIM—improves sexual vitality.

There are also mantras that relate to and improve the function of the five elements and their associated organs, states of mind, and functions . . .

LAM—earth RAM—fire HAM—ether
VAM—water YAM—air

Sanskrit syllables such as these are powerful, for the language itself is a designed spiritual language, specifically intended to bring perfect balance into life. Interestingly, the English language comes from the Celtic tree alphabet, which was equally rich and spiritually based. The fullness of the original language has been lost over time, but many of the sounds still have a powerful effect. For example, take the sound of your own name. Sing it to yourself, emphasizing each syllable. Do you identify with it? Does it please you? Does it help you to feel good about yourself? Would another name do better? Many women, particularly in the New Age movement, are changing their names as they feel the power of a new offering they can make to the world as they move into their own inherent strength. This is a recognized tradition in the east where people are frequently given new names as they progress along their spiritual path. The name itself is considered to have a transformative power.

Today, sound technology has not only transformed our music, it is also being used to enhance human functioning. One example is the Genesis, a consciousness raising sound device developed by Michael Bradford. Bradford has designed an artificially-intelligent computer that reads body rhythms and signals and will re-equalize any music being played to create the maximum enhancement of Alpha and Theta brain wave functioning. This machine is attempting to do what the Rishis of Ayurveda did when they uncovered the effects of sounds, specific mantras, and instrumentation on the human body and psyche. Bradford's device is truly Ayurvedic as it attempts to tailor its effects in accordance with our individuality.

In this day and age, we are given the opportunity to choose from the songs and traditions of the ancients or the pioneers of new technology whose consciousness and intent is to tap into that which the ancients knew and used in their own times. The choice is ours. Whichever forms we chose, take time with music. Take the time to bring beauty into your life with sound. It is another way to know yourself, nurturing yourself and making you a more beautiful person to be around.

GEMS AND JEWELRY

Gems and precious metals are used in Ayurveda to balance planetary influences and to act directly on life force. Having the capacity to both attract and dispel positive or negative energies, their healing energies are received through wearing them in jewelry or having them in some way close to the body; placing them in water overnight and drinking the water the next day; drinking water from vessels made of specific metals such as gold, silver, or copper, or taking gem tinctures in water. In the case of metal drinking vessels, gold is good for Vata while silver is good for both Pitta and Kapha. Ayurveda also uses oxidized and purified precious stones and metals in medicines. Called "basmas", these substances go deep into the body and can help in the healing of deep-seated illness or in rejuvenation. In the Ayurvedic world, Tibetans are renowned for making these precious healing substances.

If gems are to be used for healing, they should be purified by bathing them in salt water for at least two days. Water from sacred places is also sometimes used, such as water from the Ganges, the Chalice Well of Glastonbury, etc. Their power can also be increased by chanting sacred syllables and mantras over them.

The following are classifications of how gems can be most appropriately used. Choose them in accordance with what is best for you physically, mentally, and spiritually and you will—no doubt—find ones that bring out your inner beauty.

Ayurvedic Listing of Stones Useful According to Birthday

January	Garnet
February	Amethyst
March	Bloodstone
April	Diamond
May	Agate
June	Pearl
July	Ruby
August	Sapphire
September	Moonstone
October	Opal
November	Topaz
December	Ruby

In some cases it may not be possible or affordable to have one of the stones that is precious, hence costly and rare. For the above birthday list and for the lists offered below, here is a list of alternative, semi-precious stones that can be substituted . . .

Precious Stone	Semi-Precious Alternative
Ruby	Garnet
Pearl	Moonstone
Emerald	Jade or Peridot
Yellow Sapphire	Citrine
Yellow Topaz	Citrine
Diamond	Clear Zircon or Quartz
Sapphire	Amethyst

More specific recommendations come from Vedic astrological readings. Here, stones are selected to strengthen weak areas in the chart or effect healing during a certain period of time.

Gems and Doshas

First, we shall look at individual stones and how they influence the doshas . . .

Agate—decreases Kapha. Helps in protection from fear and assists in spiritual awakening.

Amethyst—decreases Vata and Pitta. Helps to balance the emotions and promotes a sense of dignity, love, compassion, and hope.

Beryl—decreases Vata and Kapha. Facilitates expression of intelligence, power, and prestige.

Diamond—White or colorless diamond stimulates Vata and Pitta and calms Kapha. Blue diamond calms Pitta and stimulates Kapha. Red diamond stimulates Pitta and encourages subtle vibrations to the heart, brain, and deep tissues. The rejuvenating effect enhances the aura and brings beauty and charm. It also helps to deepen relationships.

Lapis Lazuli—Decreases Vata and Kapha. Aids in strengthening eyes, body, and mind. Useful in spiritual practice.

Moonstone—Decreases Pitta and Vata and increases Kapha. Has a calming influence on the mind. Relieves emotional stress (also good for PMS).

Opal—Positive influence for both Vata and Kapha. Promotes friendship, compassion, creativity, and understanding.

Pearl—Decreases Vata and Pitta and increases Kapha. Calms the body and mind and is healing, especially for skin. Purifies the blood and improves vitality.

Red Coral—Decreases Vata and Pitta and increases Kapha. Purifies the blood and helps in the control of anger, jealousy, and hatred. Improves stamina and courage.

Ruby—Decreases Vata and Kapha. Improves concentration, mental power. Strengthens the will and independence.

Topaz—Decreases Vata. Helps to relieve fear.

Yellow Sapphire—Enhances energy and vitality and is generally good for health, regardless of dosha dominance.

Blue Sapphire—Helps with weight loss and has calming influence on the emotions.

As jewelry, gems are most effective when they are more than two carats and worn in contact with the skin. If you cannot get a precious stone ring or necklace of two carats or more, it is better to go with a semi-precious stone that is larger. To be in contact with the skin implies that all rings and pendants (if they are inlaid settings) should be open-backed. In all cases of the jewelry that will be mentioned with the various gems for the doshas, the preferred setting is gold unless otherwise specified.

Gems for Vata

General: (single gems) emerald, jade, peridot, yellow sapphire, topaz, garnet, ruby

(In combination with precious metals) citrine in gold, amethyst on gold necklace, beryl in silver ring worn on left ring finger

Specific: lapis lazuli on gold necklace, opal ring on right index finger, opal necklace, pearl on right ring finger, ruby on left ring finger, topaz on right index finger, topaz in necklace, yellow sapphire on index finger, blue sapphire on middle finger, moonstone in silver ring setting on right ring finger

Gems for Pitta

General: (single gems) moonstone, clear quartz, emerald, jade, pearl, peridot, blue sapphire

(in combination with precious metals) amethyst in silver, diamond in white gold ring on middle or little finger

Specific: (all in silver settings) moonstone in ring on right ring finger, pearl in ring on right ring finger, red coral ring on index finger, blue sapphire ring on middle finger

Gems for Kapha

General: (single gems) garnet, ruby, blue sapphire, amethyst

(in combination with precious metals) catseye set in gold, lapis lazuli in gold necklace with warmer stones, agate on gold necklace, beryl ring on left ring finger

Specific: diamond ring on right ring finger, opal ring on right index finger, blue sapphire ring on middle finger, ruby in silver ring on left ring finger

Explore your perfumes, experiment with new colors, buy a piece of special jewelry, and fill your life with beautiful sound.

Enjoy it all and offer the beauty you have discovered back to the world.

BENEFITS OF AYURVEDIC MASSAGE

"The secret of youth and beauty is the proper
circulation of vital life fluids and the
regular discharge of waste materials."
Harish Johari

Nothing helps the body to do just what Harish Johari says as much as massage. In fact, in the Ayurvedic tradition, massage is considered just as essential to health and beauty as good diet and other lifestyle habits. For many Indian people, massage is a regular part of a daily routine from their first day of life until their last. Babies are massaged daily until three years or so, then at least twice a week until six years of age. At six, they are encouraged to massage older members of their family in exchange for receiving massage. It is truly a family affair. Massage is given to both bride and groom before their wedding, after which they massage each other at least weekly to help shed the stress of everyday life. Women and their newborns are given daily massage for forty days after delivery. And so the circle of nurturing touch carries on. What a wonderful tradition! No wonder Indian women are known for their natural grace and charm.

Most of us in today's modern Westernized world do not have a simple way of life with the benefits of an extended family. Still, we can help ourselves using massage. It is particularly beneficial in cool climates and for those people who work more with their minds than their bodies.

Other than the obvious benefits of feeling good and being very relaxing, what else can a good massage do?

• Massage gives a beautiful lustre to the skin.

• Massage tones and relaxes the underlying muscle tissue, nourishing the skin and giving the body pleasant curves

• Massage increases body heat and improves circulation

• Massage increases the flow of life-giving oxygen to the tissues.

• Massage flushes out waste products throughout the body.

• Massage increases the body's resistance to disease by improving immune responses.

• Massage makes the body feel light, active, and energetic.

• Massage removes stiffness from the joints, improving posture and grace of movement.

• Massage makes the spine supple, improving nerve supply to the organs and all parts of the body.

• Massage increases stamina and sexual vitality.

• Massage corrects the flow of electromagnetic energy throughout the body.

• Massage improves concentration and intelligence.

• Massage builds body awareness, self-confidence, and will power.

• Massage is rejuvenating and preserves youthful qualities.

In short, massage can help keep you feeling young, vital, beautiful, and healthy. So try to get a massage as often as you can. If you cannot receive a massage for the whole body, then at least try to massage your feet on a daily basis and the head every three days or so. You can follow the instructions for a general massage of these areas as found in the overall body self-massage. At the end of this chapter, however, you will find instructions for in-depth massage procedures for the feet and, if you work a lot with your hands, a full in-depth massage for the hands.

Here follows a traditional full-body Ayurvedic massage that you can do for yourself. Try them all and fit them into your daily schedule as best you can. The benefits of such practices come quickly, so you'll be inspired and have the energy to keep going.

AYURVEDIC SELF MASSAGE TECHNIQUE

Ideally, the self massage sequence given below is done daily before a warm bath early in the morning. Many people have more time for this leisurely process in the evening. Do it when you are not rushed and have at least twenty minutes to lay down and rest before resuming normal activity.

Preparation

Warm a quarter of a cup of cold pressed sesame oil (or any oils appropriate to your dosha dominance, with or without herbal extracts or essential oils). The easiest way is to put the oil into a plastic squeezy bottle and then hold it submerged in hot water until it is pleasantly warm to the skin. (NOTE: Keep unused oil refrigerated)

Next, relax. Take some deep breaths, then rub your palms together until they feel warm. This charges the hands with energy and makes them pleasant to touch.

Massage of the Head

Pour oil on the point that is on a central hair parting, eight finger widths above your eyebrows (anterior fontanelle point). Massage the oil down both sides of the scalp towards the ears as if shampooing. Next, pour oil on the central crown point (3 finger widths behind the anterior fontanelle point) and again massage the oil into the scalp towards the ears. Tilting the head forward, pour oil onto the point where the back of the skull meets the top of the neck and rub the oil along the sides of the scalp towards the back of the ears. The whole scalp should now be oily.

Use both fists to gently tap the head all over. This stimulates the circulation and alerts the nervous system. Next, allow your fingers to rub along the scalp to get small tufts of hair and give a gentle pull on the hair from the roots. This helps relieve muscle tension that keeps the head feeling tight. In particular, be sure to pull the hair over the three points where you initially poured the oil. (Diagram 1)

Clockwise motion is generally favored for massage as it releases tension. It is always used on marma points to strengthen and enrich the body.

 Anticlockwise motion 'stirs up' energy in the body. It is used more rarely, never on marma points, and usually follwed by clock-wise massage.

These lines on the front and back of the leg show where to apply oil, stroking against the direction of hair growth.

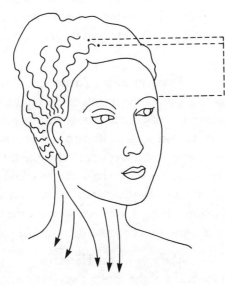

CROWN POINT

3 finger widths behind anterior fontanelle

8 finger widths above eyebrows

Diagram 1. Self massage of the head and neck

Massage of the Face

Keeping the fingertips well oiled, do massage strokes from the central portion of the forehead (above and between the eyebrows) outward toward the hair line on both sides of the face. Continue to stroke over every contour of the face, from the midline of the face outward and upward; over the forehead, above and below each eye, along the cheeks from the nose, above and below the lips and be sure to include underneath the chin and up under the jaw. Tap under the chin and pinch along the jaw.

Massage of the Neck

(Remember to keep hands well oiled from here on so they can slide easily over the body. Generously oil all joints in the area you are focusing on.)

Using all four fingers together, stroke up the back of the neck; use the right hand for the left side of the neck and vice versa. Stroke down both sides of the front of the neck, avoiding direct pressure on the windpipe. Generally, the rule is to use strokes up the back of the body (thus up the back of the neck) and down the front (thus down front of the neck).

Massage of the Arms

Using the palms and all of the fingers of the right hand to work on the left arm first, use small circular strokes to vigorously massage the shoulders, elbows, and wrist joints. Stroke down the muscles of the front or inside upper and lower arm, following the contours of the muscles. Then continue up the back on the outside of the arm in one motion. Working along the natural curves and shapes of the muscles in this manner is most relaxing. Now use the left hand for the right arm and repeat the sequence. (Diagram 2, pps. 128-129)

Massage of the Hands

Stroke down the backs of the hands, then down each finger in a milking, pulling action. Using the thumb of the opposite hand, smooth out the palm, starting at the heel of the hand and working over the palm toward the base of the fingers. Repeat for opposite hand.

Massage of the Trunk

Using the flat of the hands, massage in large circles over the whole front of the body moving upwards and outwards from the body's midline. Start at the shoulder and work over the chest to the bottom of the ribs. Massage the abdomen in circles, spiralling out from the belly button in a clockwise direction (upwards starting on the right, across the upper abdomen, down to the left and across from left to right below the navel).

Massage the back as best you can, starting at the base of the spine, working upward and outward from the backbone out over the ribs. To complete, squeeze the tops of the shoulders. (Diagram 2, pps. 128-129)

Massage of the Legs

Massage the buttocks with large clockwise circular strokes. Apply oil to the whole leg, stroking upwards against the direction of hair growth so the oil is absorbed well. Using both hands, one on the inside and one on the outside of the leg, massage down the front of the leg, starting at hip and drawing the hands towards the midline of the front of the thigh, stroking inward and downwards. For the back of the upper leg, start just above either side of the knee and stroke inwards and upwards towards the midline of the back of the thigh. Start with the right leg first.

Stroke down the front of the lower legs from the knee to the ankle and up the back of the leg, starting from the ankle and working up the calf to the back of the knee in the same manner you did the upper leg. (Diagram 2, pps. 128-129)

Stroke down the foot and pull on the toes in a similar manner as you did your fingers. Pay particular attention to the arch of your foot and top of your foot at the base of the top of the toes. Massage the soles of the feet with a generous amount of oil, making sure you rub both feet equally well. The foot reflexology chart provided will help you locate areas on the soles of the feet that correspond to the organs and structure of the body. Gently rub any areas that are sore. Always finish with a gentle circular rub to the kidney areas. (Diagram 7, p. 137)

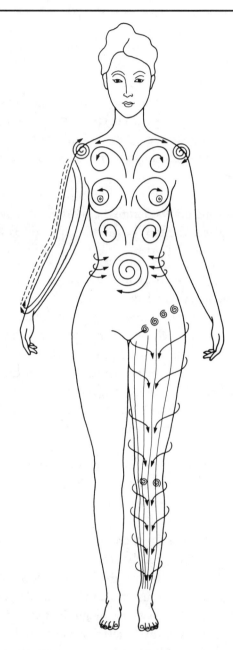

Diagram 2. Self massage of the front of the body
note: strokes are basically downward

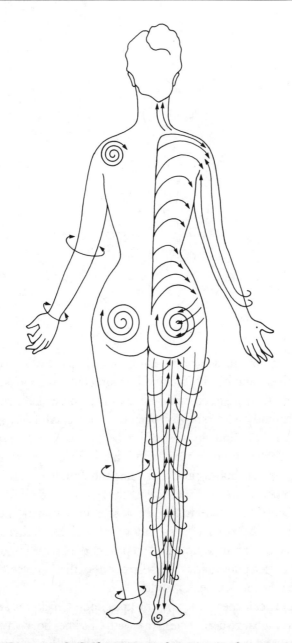

Diagram 2. Self massage of the back of the body
note: strokes are basically upward around and over joints

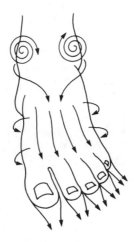

Diagram 3 (Foot Massage)

Complete your massage by putting a few drops of warm sesame oil in each ear and nostril, the navel, around the anus and genitals.

After the massage, rest a while. Have a small nourishing snack and take a pleasantly warm shower to remove the excess oil. Use a paste made of chickpea flour and water or milk applied just before rinsing off or while the water is not running. This does a fine job of removing the excess oil, buffing and energizing the skin. In contrast, soap scours deeper, temporarily destroying the skin's mantle. This mantle is the body's first barrier to undesirable substances entering the body via the skin. The soap may also remove some of the oil that should be allowed to remain to nourish and protect the body. If you must use a soap, use a pure, mild castile soap or one of the Ayurvedic soaps available (See the Source Appendix).

About the chickpea paste and chickpea flour: Chickpeas are also known as Garbanzo beans here in the West. Chickpea flour is available at oriental and Indian markets, where it is called "fine Graham" or

"Besan" flour. Chickpea flour that is available at health food stores is generally too coarse for the purpose of using it on the skin. Chickpea paste to be used in one's shower is made by mixing eight (8) heaping tablespoons (English dessert spoons) with half a cup of milk or water. Apply this paste sparingly over your body while in the bath or shower stall. Rub gently, then rinse it off. If you do not wish to make this paste, you can, alternatively, sprinkle dry Chickpea Flour directly on your body and briskly rub it over the skin surface. Allow the flour to stay on your body for a minute or so in order for it to absorb some of the excess oil from your pores. Then rinse with warm water. Both methods leave the skin smooth, soft, and tinglingly fresh.

After your rinse—if you want to be a little more luxurious, add milk powder or essential oils to a warm bath and soak up the goodness. Milk naturally softens and nourishes the skin while essential oils help relax both the mind and body. See the section on *Aroma, Colors, and Gems* for recipes most appropriate for your constitution and condition.

If you have used a generous amount of oil on your head, you will need to shampoo thoroughly.

IN-DEPTH HAND AND FOOT MASSAGE TECHNIQUES
(The following hand and foot massage techniques can be used in conjunction with the full body massage or alone.)

Hand Massage
Hand massage works deeply by stimulating acupuncture points and energy meridians that run through the hands to the tips of the fingers. And, like foot reflexology, the hand has areas that are associated with the various organs and systems within the body. If you try massaging these specific areas, work gently and for short periods at first. Be sure to do similar points on both hands and always end by gently stimulating the kidney area in the center of the palm. This helps the body deal more easily with the extra toxins that you release through the hand massage. (Diagram 5, p. 134)

It is better not to work on specific areas during pregnancy as toxins can be released into the developing fetus and cause weakness.

1) Apply a few drops of warm oil to the center of the palm. Using the thumb of the opposite hand, start from the heel of the hand and firmly stroke up towards the fingers, starting outwards towards the base of the index finger, then each finger in turn, finishing with the little finger. Pay attention to those special reflexology areas on the palm.

2) Massage at the base of each of the fingers in small circles and then on the sides of the palm.

3) Turning the hand over, massage between the ligaments on the back of the hand from the wrist into the webs between the fingers. Press and massage the spot between the thumb and index finger as indicated in the diagram. This helps digestion and can relieve headaches.

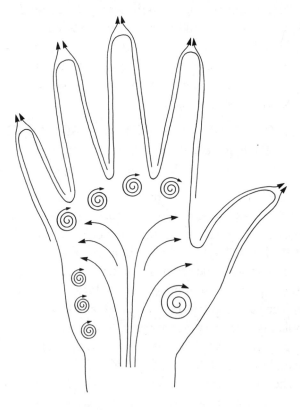

Diagram 4 (Palm)

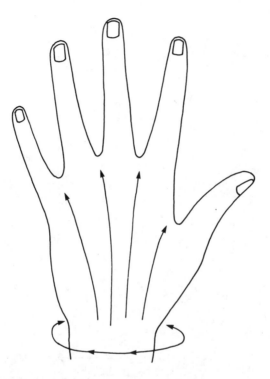

Diagram 4 (Back)

4) Working on the thumb and fingers . . . starting with the thumb, pinch from the base to the tip on the front and back and along both sides. Next do the index finger like this and work your way to the little finger. Repeat this several times, making a point to pay attention to and work thoroughly over and around all of the joints in the fingers and thumb. After perhaps three times you should feel a free flow of energy moving through the fingers.

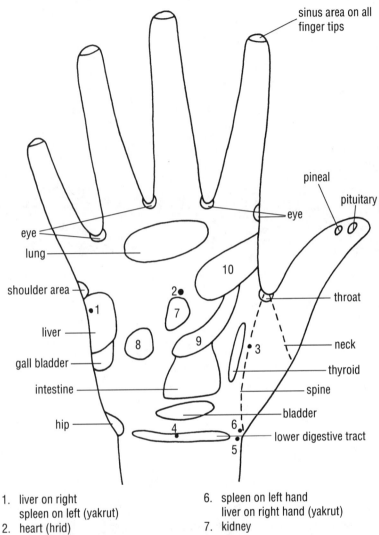

sinus area on all finger tips

pineal

pituitary

eye

eye

lung

shoulder area

throat

liver

neck

gall bladder

thyroid

intestine

spine

hip

bladder

lower digestive tract

1. liver on right
   spleen on left (yakrut)
2. heart (hrid)
3. digestive point on palm
   sinus point on back of hand (talus)
4-5 massage to strengthen entire body
   (manibandha)

6. spleen on left hand
   liver on right hand (yakrut)
7. kidney
8. pancreas
9. colon
10. stomach

HAND MASSAGE
Reflex areas and Marma points

Diagram 5

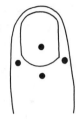

Diagram 6

5) Press each of the points shown in the finger nail diagram on each of the fingers. Press, then quickly release. Do this several times.

6) To complete the hand massage, rub them together palm to palm, then palm to the back of the hand and let them rest.

This is actually a very vigorous process. It makes you work in a small area with a lot of attention. If there is pain or stiffness in the hands from doing this, you can condition your hands with Chinese iron balls. These balls are a fun and gentle way to exercise and strengthen your hands.

Foot Massage *(Padabhyanga):*
"Diseases do not go near one who massages his feet before sleeping just as snakes do not approach eagles."
Ancient Indian Saying

According to tradition, beauty in the body arises from a straight, strong back. Healthy nerves from the spine provide quality stimulation to all the organs and allow for graceful movement. But, for us to carry ourselves out into the world in a graceful manner, we also need strong, beautiful feet to support our steps and ground our energy.

As with the hands and ears, touching the soles of the feet stimulates, cleanses, and balances all of the organs in the body. This is one good reason for going barefoot regularly. There is nothing more wonderful than walking on a pebbly beach or running through grass covered in morning dew. That is why intentionally massaging the soles of the feet is relaxing.

Massage of the feet prevents and cures dryness, numbness, roughness, fatigue, and cracking of the heels. It strengthens walking and running. Foot Reflexology, a healing art that specifically focuses on the feet as being a reflection of all the organs and structures in the entire body, is wonderful for relieving acute pain, improving posture, as well as health of the organs. According to the Ayurvedic physician, Vagbhata, nerves in the soles of the feet are connected to the eyes and ears. Thus, massage to the feet can help with the functioning of these sense organs. A good massage before bed can ensure a restful night's sleep.

As with the hands, work gently and for short periods of time on the specific points of the feet, working on the same areas of both feet. Use oils in accordance with needs and conditions. Generally, use sesame oil. Sesame and brahmi oils promote deep refreshing sleep. (You'll need to wear socks to keep the sheets clean until the oil is absorbed.) Mustard oil protects the feet from the drying effects of cold weather and also helps prevent the growth of athlete's foot. Essential oils of lavender and rosemary, added to the base oil, are wonderful for active legs (refer to Diagram 3, p. 130).

• **Massage the Ankle**— Rub oil vigorously into the whole ankle joint, emphasizing the areas around the bones on the inner and outer side of the ankle. Pinch down the large (Achilles) tendon that connects the calf muscle to the heel. Repeat this stroking and kneading of this tendon several times.

• **Massage the Top of the Foot**— Supporting the foot by holding the heel and letting the arch rest on the palm, use the thumb of the other hand to firmly stroke from the ankle between the tendons to between each of the toes. Repeat twice.

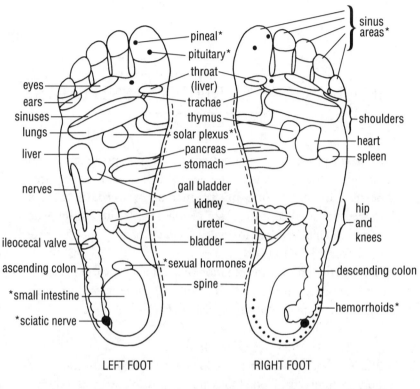

sinus areas*

pineal*

pituitary*

throat (liver)

eyes

ears

sinuses

lungs

liver

trachae

thymus

solar plexus*

pancreas

stomach

shoulders

heart

spleen

nerves

gall bladder

kidney

ureter

bladder

hip and knees

ileocecal valve

ascending colon

*small intestine

*sciatic nerve

*sexual hormones

spine

descending colon

hemorrhoids*

LEFT FOOT

RIGHT FOOT

* mirrored on other foot

Diagram 7 (Foot Massage)

• **Massage the Toes**—Starting with the big toe and ending with the baby toe pinch from the base on either side to the tip of the toes. Pull and rotate each toe, massaging on all sides. Oil well between the toes.
• **Massage Reflexively on the Soles**—referring to a foot reflex chart, work on the head and neck areas, the shoulder, the spine, then any problem area, ending with the kidneys. (Please note that reflexive foot massage is not advised during pregnancy.)

SPECIAL CARE OF REGIONS AND PARTS OF THE BODY

Ayurveda emphasizes self-knowledge and appropriate self care to keep the body both inwardly and outwardly beautiful and healthy. The traditional role of a practitioner of Ayurveda is to be a knowledgeable guide; to educate people in self-care and provide medicines or interventions to bring individuals back to a point where self-care can be continued.

Towards this end, the information that follows provides a guide to preventive care for specific regions and parts of the body together with some home remedies for simple disorders.

The Mouth

Efficient digestion and elimination are central to both health and beauty in Ayurveda. Good looks are not possible without optimal functioning of digestion and elimination.

The mouth is the first organ of digestion, being the first place where food enters the body. Chewing well and thoroughly tasting food is essential to efficient digestion. Good chewing goes a long way to compensating for not eating foods that are best for you and it also ensures that when you eat quality food, you are getting the most from it. To chew well, strong teeth and healthy gums are needed. To taste foods properly you need a strong, clean tongue and a good sense of smell.

To help keep the teeth strong, clean and floss them morning and evening. Brush them with herbal or Ayurvedic tooth preparations. These products usually taste good, are fresher for the breath, and will help strengthen both teeth and gums. Use a soft nylon or natural bristle brush. Brush teeth away from the gums or in tiny circles and make sure to reach all surfaces of the teeth. On a preventive note, limit or avoid soft drinks, sucking candy or chewing sweet things that stick to your teeth—even raisins. They not only erode the protective enamel of the teeth, but leech precious minerals out of the body, weakening teeth and bones in general. After they are ingested, foods that are high in minerals strengthen the teeth. Sea vegetables, dark greens, and quality dairy foods help strengthen teeth from within.

Healthy teeth need healthy gums to hold them in position and supply nutrients. Flossing helps bleeding gums by removing trapped food particles and tartar build-up. Gum massage is also very helpful. Try to massage the gums daily, especially if they show signs of receding. Here is a simple, but useful recipe for a gum massage mixture:

5 parts alum powder (helps to tighten gums)

2 parts rock salt (soothes)

3 parts black pepper (disinfects)

1 part turmeric (tightens gums, increases blood flow and disinfects)

Use this mixture as a powder or mix with a little sesame oil, clove oil, or ghee for easier application. Use the middle finger and massage the gums in small, anti-clockwise circles. For those of you who are not attracted to this procedure, you might try the advice of a British dentist and a student of Ayurveda: Massage the gums with a mashed strawberry. It does a great job of cleaning the teeth and it's astringent qualities tone the gums.

The tongue is the mirror for the condition of the intestines. Coating on the tongue shows a presence of ama or undigested toxic material in the digestive tract (as well as not being very attractive). This coating is a discharge, like urine or sweat and needs to be removed each morning lest it is swallowed back down into the system when eating and drinking. Scrape the tongue using a silver, copper, or stainless steel spoon or an Ayurvedic tongue scraper, available through suppliers of Ayurvedic products. Be gentle, especially if the tongue is inflamed. A coating towards the back of the tongue suggests a problem in the large intestine; the middle has more to do with the stomach and small intestine. Improving digestion will cure a sticky, thickly coated tongue over time. This takes longest for Vata constitution as Vata digestion is so variable. Tongue diagnosis is as complex as pulse taking, but some simple explanations are given in Dr. Vasant Lad's *Ayurveda: the Science of Self-Healing.*

Regarding bad breath, for a full cure seek to improve digestion. Try a half cup of aloe vera juice twice a day. Also, chew roasted fennel seeds after meals. Both of these techniques are symptomatic and help the digestive process.

The Throat

Gargle each day to clear mucous from the throat using a pinch of salt and turmeric in a cup of warm water. To sooth a sore throat, gargle with the herbal infusion (found below), chew licorice root or slowly lick a spoon of honey. The herbal infusion is soothing and anti-bacterial. Licorice clears congestion and soothes pain. Honey is a strong anti-bacterial agent.

Gargle Infusion:

1 tspn. sage

1 tspn. dried plantain

1 tspn. dried rosemary

1 tspn. dried honeysuckle

Infuse in 1 pint of water. Use honey for more taste.

The salt and turmeric gargle mentioned earlier is also useful for sore throat.

Ears

Each morning, use your little finger to apply a drop or two of sesame oil around the opening of the ear canal. This helps keep Vata dosha in balance, oil is always calming to Vata, and maintains good hearing. It also helps to reduce jaw tension.

Massage of the ears benefits the whole body, reducing fatigue and freshening the senses. Gently pull the ear flaps down and then back, then up and back again. Rub them with your full hand until they tingle. (Flicking your ears back and forth in very cold weather is a way of generating heat in the body.)

Once each month or more often if you are in very Vata deranging situations, have someone give you *karna purana*. This is an Ayurvedic process that fills the ear to the fullness of the canal with warm sesame oil. For details of the procedure, check the special treatments section. This helps with jaw tension, ringing in the ears, earaches, headaches, teeth and gum disorders, even burning sensation in the feet. Do this procedure early in the day before eating.

The Nose

The nose is called the door to the brain, possibly because brain function is so strongly influenced by smell.

As you did with the ears, each morning, use your little finger to apply a little sesame oil or ghee around the inside of each nostril. This helps one to maintain a keen sense of smell and calms the mind by helping to keep Vata dosha in balance. Massaging the tip of the nose stimulates the heart while massaging the flare of the nose stimulates the lungs.

Washing the sinus passages using clean, warm water with a pinch of salt and a pinch of turmeric is a common practice in India. It may be done daily or whenever the sinuses are congested with mucous, clogged from inhaling dust and dirt, or dry and inflamed. Gently inhale the mixture up one nostril at a time. Allow the mix to drain into the back of your mouth and then spit it out. Repeat on the other side. Getting water up the nostrils is most efficiently done using an Ayurvedic *neti* pot. However, a cup will do. For clearing the nasal passages and other medicinal purposes, *nasya* is also performed. See details of this procedure in the section on special Ayurvedic treatments.

Eyes

Being Pitta in nature, the eyes benefit from being kept cool. Wash them gently with water no hotter than body temperature. Water that has been held in the mouth will be the correct temperature and that little bit of saliva that is mixed in it will act as a natural bacteriostatic.

For dry or itchy eyes and for general benefit to eyesight, place a drop of sesame oil in each eye. As this will initially mist over the vision, it is most convenient to do this directly before sleeping. The special Ayurvedic procedure of *netra basti* is also excellent to take for these conditions.

For tense or bloodshot eyes, use a couple of drops of pure rose water to soothe the eyes as necessary or once a week for prevention. On a daily basis, rest with your eyes. You may cover them with slices of cool cucumber, or cotton balls soaked in aloe vera, cilantro juice, eyebright or fennel tea. Interestingly, oiling the soles of the feet with castor oil also pulls heat from the eyes. Honey, castor oil, barberry, or triphala tea applications may be used under the direction of an Ayurvedic practitioner to remedy simple eye complaints.

In general, factors that damage the eyes include:
- studying in improper or inadequate light
- watching a lot of or being close up to a T.V.
- staring at computer screens for long periods
- being in overly bright light
- looking at solar eclipses without proper precautions
- heating the head
- using hot water to wash the hair
- eating very spicy food and drink

To improve eyesight:
- reduce hours spent in artificial light
- use full spectrum lighting for both regular incandescent and fluorescent lights
- gaze at a flame of a butter lamp or candle for 20 minutes daily

- massage and oil your big toes
- do eye exercises

Television and computer screens are very stressful for the eyes. They also heat the eyes. *Netra basti* or the treatment of having ghee in the eyes for a period of time is very useful. One way you can do this treatment for yourself is to use an old pair of swimming goggles and pour warm ghee into each eye cup. Place the cups against the eyes securely and lean back on something that it will not matter if a little ghee drips onto it. Allow the eyes to roll around in this warm ghee for about ten minutes. Lean forward to allow the ghee to drain back in the cups.

The Hands

My mother has always said that a woman's hands give away her age quicker than her face. Just doing everyday jobs, the hands are in contact with chemicals, detergents, and various forms of filth and dirt that damage the skin and bring about premature aging.

To treat them kindly, wear protective gloves for doing the dishes and other work that involves direct contact with these substances. Massage them regularly with hand cream. If you don't like to wear gloves while working, try this protective hand cream recipe . . .

1 egg yolk
1 Tablespoon of marigold oil
kaolin (or fine clay) powder to mix.

Mix the egg yolk and marigold oil with enough kaolin powder to make a paste. Rub into your hands. Do your work and then rinse the mixture off when you are done. This is particularly helpful in protecting your hands from gritty and ground in dirt.

To protect and nourish hard-working hands, use the following lotion:

3 Tablespoons lanolin
1 Tablespoon ghee
6 Tablespoons sesame oil

10 drops chamomile essential oil or one of your choice

Use this somewhat thick lotion. If you would like to make this lighter, decrease the lanolin and increase the oil.

When hands are strong, healthy, and well cared for, they have a natural energy that is felt even in the most casual hand shake. Take care of your hands and you will communicate strength and love to whomever you touch.

Nail Care

The fingernails are the by-product (mala) of the *asthi dhatu* (bones). Each dhatu is inter-related as they nourish each other in a sequential fashion. This means that the condition of the nails reflects the condition of all body tissues up to *majja* and *shukra dhatus* and their related *upadhatus* and *malas*. The solutions for problems with the nails, then, have to address the balance and nourishment of the whole system.

Conditions of the Nails:

• Horizontal indentations indicate a derangement in agni—a weakening in the digestive capacity. Thus agni is what needs to be addressed. Solutions to problems with agni can be found on page 50.

• Vertical ridges show long-standing Vata derangement. This often means a weakened digestion that does not metabolize minerals or proteins well and a deficiency in Vitamin B12 and Iron.

• White spots show a calcium or zinc deficiency. They often appear after a period of eating sweets, especially refined sugars that leech minerals out of the body.

• Bitten nails show nervousness, mineral deficiency, or intestinal parasites—generally a high Vata condition.

• Hang nails show a lack of protein, Vit. C, and folic acid in the body due to low intake of these nutrients or poor absorption.

• Brittle nails show low iron or Vitamin A, imbalanced thyroid or kidney function and poor circulation.

• Split nails show low agni in the stomach.

• Reddish purple nails show weakening of the body and general fatigue.
• Dark red nails show blood stagnation due to eating heavy, salty, fatty foods.
• Yellowish nails show liver imbalance.
• Bluish nails show lung and heart imbalance.
• Pale nails show poor blood condition, anemia, and low liver and kidney energy.

The condition of the nails is not only influenced by the blood quality and nourishment from the other dhatus, but also by the electro-magnetic energy that flows through the body in the system of meridians. If a particular nail has problems, look for a corresponding imbalance in the organ whose meridian is associated with that finger and nail.
• Thumb nail is an indicator for the brain.
• Index finger nail is an indicator for the lungs and colon.
• Middle finger nail is an indicator for the small intestine.
• Ring finger nail is an indicator for the kidney.
• Little finger nail is an indicator for the heart and female reproductive organs.

Following a diet and lifestyle that is suitable for your body type and condition is then a key to beautiful nails. The diet should be rich in proteins and nail building minerals such as sulphur, calcium, iron, silica, zinc, as well as essential fatty acids and vitamins like biotin, vitamin D, and Vitamins A and E. Check the diet section for sources of these nutrients.

Healthy nails are pinkish in color, smooth, and evenly shaped. The actual shape and consistency varies with which dosha is dominant. Vata-type nails tend to be the most irregular in shape and are prone to being pale and brittle. Pitta nails are an even oval shape, soft, flexible, and pink. Kapha nails are squarer, thick, and strong.

Like the skin and hair, healthy nails rely on their growth areas or roots being well nourished and efficiently cleansed. Nail care follows the familiar pattern of cleansing, then nourishing.

The same procedures to be described here can also be applied to the toe nails.

On a daily basis, use a soft nail brush to clean and massage the nails and finger tips. This not only cleans, but stimulates circulation. Rubbing the finger nails of both hands together (i.e. against each other) charges the body's energy meridians. It is also said to promote hair growth.

Once a week give your nails a little extra care. Soak your nails in warm water and lemon juice. Take your fingertips out of the solution and gently scrub them with a brush. Soak again briefly, then pat dry. Now massage each nail with sesame or a medicated oil. Neem oil nourishes and strengthens the nails while lemon oil is good for dry, brittle nails. For the fingers and nails, follow steps 4 and 5 in the Hand Massage procedure (pps. 133 & 135).

A natural smoothness and shine can be brought to the nails by bathing them in warm vegetable oil with a few drops of added essential oils.

General Nail Care formula:
1 oz. almond oil
2 drops lavender oil
2 drops sandalwood oil
2 drops cypress oil

Feet and Foot Care

Although foot massage is quite beneficial, simply bathing the feet can freshen and revive the whole system. In hot dusty countries like India, bathing the hands, face, and feet is suggested upon waking, before eating or meditating, before sleep, and whenever you would like to revive and refresh yourself, or whenever a full bath or shower is not possible.

Foot Soaks:

What follows are a variety of foot soaks or baths to help relieve, revive, and invigorate your feet. Use a bucket or bowl large enough so water can cover the feet over the ankles.

• **For Calming and Cooling**—Prepare a cool bath with a handful of sandalwood powder or a few drops of essential oil of sandalwood. This soak cools the whole body and frees the mind of the troubles of the day. It is a wonderful help for restful sleep on a hot summer's night.

• **For Invigorating**—get a handful each of crushed juniper berries, rosemary, and lavender. Brew these in a pint of boiling water, strain after 10 minutes and add to a hot foot bath.

• **For Deodorizing**—Place a small handful of sage, thyme, lavender, sweet marjoram, bay leaf, and a tablespoon of rock salt and brew them in one pint of boiling water. Strain and add to a warm foot bath. Leaving the herbs in will create a stronger smell for deodorizing.

• **For a Thick Head Cold**—Prepare a hot foot bath with a handful or two of ginger or mustard powder. Grated fresh ginger or ginger essential oil can also be used. Leave the feet in the solution until they are bright red. Pat dry and put on warm socks. This procedure warms the whole body and drains mucous and congestion from the head.

• **For Burning Hot Feet**—For this condition, use a poultice of henna leaf powder and vinegar or lemon juice. (Beware—Henna will dye your skin orange. Orange palms and soles of the feet are a common sight in India and North Africa.) Also, massaging the feet with bhringaraj oil is also very cooling.

• **For a Sound and Restful Sleep**— Massage the feet with warm sesame oil or ghee. Then soak the feet in a hot herbal foot bath prepared with warming herbs and spices, such as ginger.

• **Healing the Skin**—Try a warm foot bath prepared with strongly brewed marigold.

• **For Hard Skin**—Massage the feet with sesame oil, then submerge them in a hot foot bath of mustard or ginger tea solution. Prepare the solution by mixing a small teaspoon of ginger or mustard powder in one pint of boiling water. Add to the bath. Allow the feet to get bright red, then scrub them with a loofa or pumice stone. (For cracked heels, massage in a paste of nutmeg and milk or apply a castor oil poultice.)

• **For Sweaty Feet**—Submerge your feet in warm water with equal amounts of essential oils of lavender and sage or clary sage, juniper, and cypress. Use 6 to 9 drops per 2½ pints of water.

• **For Tired Feet**—Use a foot bath that has juniper, rosemary, and lavender essential oils mixed in. Proportions should be the same as one's given for Sweaty Feet foot bath.

• **Nature's Foot Bath**—Take an early morning barefoot walk, in cool, dewy grass. It is refreshing and nourishing for body and soul. It is a standard in Kneipp hydrotherapy and favored in macrobiotic circles as an aid to female reproductive health.

As a final note about feet, try to give them air as much as possible. As mentioned earlier, barefoot is best. However it is not always practical. At least go shoeless in your own home. Shoes trap energy around the feet and in the long run can make you feel more tired. They collect negativity which is one reason why they are never worn in Indian temples. Take them off when you can.

Hair Care

For thick, strong glossy hair the roots must be firm and the scalp healthy and well nourished. By analogy, as the skin is a rolling landscape, the hair is a tall grassland needing moisture, nourishment, and a firm root system to flourish.

Just as drought and blazing heat quickly destroys a lawn, heat is most detrimental for the hair. Too much sun dries the hair and heats the head, weakening the scalp and hair roots. My father recalls that his hair started to thin after he was given a 'crew cut' then got his head sunburnt aboard a ship bound for the Near East during World War II. So, although we have treated this story as a bit of a joke at my father's expense, it could well be that the hot Mediterranean sun damaged my father's hair roots which subsequently led to his baldness. Protect your hair by wearing a hat or head scarf when out in strong sunlight for long periods of time, especially if you are a blonde or redhead.

High Pitta heat within the body can also damage hair at the roots. Heat naturally rises and leaves the body at the crown of the head. As Pitta types naturally have the greatest amount of body heat, they are most prone to premature greying and balding. I have seen women that have large grey streaks coming from the region of their crown area. Besides high Pitta, excess heat can be generated by eating a high red meat diet. Head heat can also be generated by a lot of mental activity. Interestingly the absent-minded professor is often portrayed as bald or with wild, dry grey locks.

Both the brain and the scalp prefer to be kept cool, so even when washing the hair it is best to use warm water and a cool rinse. Cold water is more efficient at removing soap anyway as well as being toning to the scalp and refreshing to the nervous system.

A balanced diet rich in protein, minerals, and vitamins, especially iron, sulphur, zinc, B complex, and Vitamin C as well as essential fatty acids is essential for healthy hair. Just as with the skin, health comes from within. In fact, the hair so well reflects the internal state of the body that hair analysis is widely used by nutritionists and health care professionals to discover toxicity and nutritional deficiencies in clients.

Nutrients are key to healthy hair, but to be effective they must reach the roots. Often tension in the scalp or fatty deposits block circulation, drying the sebum and, thus, literally starving the hair roots. Massage is the answer for tension relief to improve circulation and freeing the hair roots of dry sebum.

A head massage is one of the most relaxing and pleasurable experiences. Massage while shampooing is good, but as with the skin, oil massage is better. Traditionally a variety of herbal oils have been used. The herbs enhance the effect of the massage by nourishing and strengthening the hair roots and promoting hair growth. The base oil is usually sesame or coconut oil. Pumpkin seed or almond oil can also be used. These are enhanced by amla, shikaikai, neem, sandalwood, jasmine, coriander, in combination or individually. However, bhringaraj or brahmi are the most commonly used herbal oils used for hair. Refer to the massage section for head massage. Also see the "massage of the head" referred to in the self-massage section.

Warm the oil before the massage, as it is more relaxing and penetrates better. Once the oil has been thoroughly massaged into the scalp, brush the hair with a natural bristle or nylon brush with little rubber rounded ends and then wrap the head in a warm towel. Leave for a minimum of twenty minutes or overnight if possible. When the body rests, the skin is more able to take in nourishment. This treatment is very nourishing to the scalp, hair roots, and the hair itself. It works as an excellent pre-wash conditioner and is the best way to combat dryness from tints, perms, electric curlers and blow drying, and promotes healthy new hair growth.

Traditionally, powdered herbs were used to cleanse the hair, lifting dirt without disturbing the natural functioning of the scalp. Such powders are available, some using Ayurvedic herbs, others western. Gentle shampoos that contain Ayurvedic extracts of neem, amla, and shikakai are also available for you to try. Please avoid shampoos that use sudsing agents such as sodium and ammonium lauryl sulphate. The foam they make has little to do with their cleansing effects. They are simple harsh chemicals that strip the outer protein layer of the hair and dry the scalp, making the use of conditioners necessary. Conditioners do little more than provide an oily film that traps dirt and makes the hair look dull. They are not necessary for healthy hair.

Dry Shampoo
    1 tspn. orris root powder
    2 tspn. arrowroot powder
    1-2 tspn. herbs (alma, neem, sandalwood)

Part hair and sprinkle in the partings. Leave for 10 minutes. Brush until all the powder is out, taking with it dirt and excess oil.

Wet Shampoo
>1 Tbl. grated or powdered soapwort
>1 handful of herbs of those used in the oils or rinses are most suitable
>½ pint boiling water

Pour boiling water over the mixture. Allow to cool, strain, and use as you would regular shampoo.

If you feel that you still need a conditioner, try this recipe:
>3 Tbl. herbal oils (as advised for head massage)
>1 Tbl. cider vinegar or fresh lemon juice
>1 egg yolk
>1 tspn. honey
>few drops of essential oils per hair condition

Perms and dyes chemically alter the shaft of the hair, often making it dry and brittle. Natural perms are now commonly available as well as more natural dying processes. Herbal hair rinses are the safest way to highlight and enhance natural hair color and bring a glossy shine as well as strength and thickness.

Natural Hair Rinses

Conditioning Rinses—Lemon juice, vinegar, or beer helps to thoroughly remove soap and conditioner residue. They swell the keratin layer making the hair glossy and smooth. An egg yolk added to the rinse gives it a natural protein and sulphur boost. Use an essential oil in the rinse as the eggy smell tends to linger. Yoghurt can be used also as it naturally softens the hair.

Lightening Rinses—Use chamomile tea, marigold tea, or onion juice to brighten blonde hair. Rhubarb root is a natural yellow hair dye. Ceylonese black tea brings out golden highlights. Use lemon juice rinse, then dry hair in the sun for a natural bleach. Remember to not let the head get too hot.

Darkening Rinses—Using rosemary, sage, bhringaraj, and brahmi rinses and oils will darken and bring luster to the hair.

For Red High Lights—Use henna powder. A large variety of natural hennas are commercially available, red through natural. Always test henna on a tiny strip of hair before using. The effect of henna can be especially strong on blonde or grey hair. The acid of lemon juice or vinegar will strengthen the dying effect. Henna mixed with black coffee or burgundy wine will make a darker, richer color.

Hair Problems

Dry Hair—Reduce factors in your lifestyle that aggravate Vata dosha. Make sure you have plenty of zinc and essential fatty acids in your diet. Give yourself regular warm oil head massages. Use amla, shikaikai, brahmi oils or warm sesame oil with essential oils of lavender, geranium, or juniper.

Oily Hair—Reduce factors in your lifestyle that aggravate Pitta dosha, especially oily foods. Wash your hair regularly, use lemony rinses, brush your hair well and don't be afraid to use oily massage. Massage helps balance the scalp condition, especially when herbal essential oils are used. Neem oil works well or jojoba oil with essential oil of bergamot, clary sage, juniper, cedarwood, cypress, lemon, and lavender.

Dandruff—This problem often resolves with a natural foods diet and improved agni. Sometimes it is aggravated by allergies or particular foods that stress the liver. These foods include heavy, fatty foods like milk, yoghurt, cheese, peanut butter, and fatty red meats. Massage helps to stimulate the scalp and circulation. Essential oils of eucalyptus and rose in jojoba oil (20 drops per 2 fluid ounces) also helps this condition. Eucalyptus stimulates and cleanses the scalp while rose tones and soothes. For itchy dandruff with flaking and inflammation, geranium, lavender, juniper, and sandalwood essential oils in combination with jojoba oil as a base is helpful. Massage well into the scalp, leave overnight, and shampoo well in the morning. Oily, scaling scalp is helped by cedar, rosemary, and lemon essential oils. Dietwise, eating parsley and using a parsley rinse also helps. Parsley is very rich in nutrients for hair and is toning and soothing to use externally.

Hair Loss—As well as a poor diet, hair can be severely damaged by many other factors. Besides external and internal heat as already mentioned, some of the other factors include:
- stress and tension that tightens the scalp and reduces circulation
- hormonal changes in pregnancy and menopause
- thyroid imbalance
- medications, especially diet pills
- illness and/or allergies
- shock or long-term worry
- over-processing with perms and dyes
- genetic tendencies

To remedy this condition, massage with bhringaraj and brahmi oils. Work deeply into the scalp to relax and nourish the nervous system, useful against all the factors listed and helps to rejuvenate the hair roots so they can once again produce healthy hair.

In New Mexico a plant called Yerba de la Negrita is used. It's action is to soften the sebum that is often dry, binding the hair roots. Once the roots are clear and healthy, the hair is free to grow. This is New Mexico Ayurveda!

Breast Care

To get a firm youthful quality to your breasts, two oils are traditionally advised. They can be prepared in the same manner as herbal massage oils. Mix together the ingredients listed below. Bring to a boil. Gently simmer until water is evaporated. Cool in refrigerator until ready to use.

Pomegranate Toner:

>   1 part powdered pomegranate rind
>   4 part mustard oil
>   16 parts water

Shatavari Ghee:

>   1 part shatavari powder
>   4 parts ghee
>   16 parts water

For best results, massage breasts with either the toner or ghee daily in the evening.

AYURVEDIC SKIN CARE

"When we take time for ourselves, it's an act of loving ourselves, and we can extend that love to our families and the world around us. We find balance and inner harmony that radiates to everyone in our lives."
Marj Campian, director
Delicious Magazine, March 1990

Very few people are blessed with naturally perfect skin. More people today are living in cities, constantly exposed to dirt and pollution, pursuing high speed, tension-producing lifestyles, yet aspiring to natural beauty! Toxins seem to be everywhere: in the food we eat, water we drink, air we breathe. With a diminishing ozone layer, even sunshine is becoming hazardous. Stress levels for women are perhaps at an all time high with competitiveness in the workplace and less well defined roles for both themselves and men. Consequently, to achieve that natural look, a regular skin care program is no longer a luxury, but an essential anxiety reliever and beauty therapy to combat the ravages of modern living.

This chapter describes cosmetics and procedures that will convert your home into a natural beauty salon or, if you own or run a salon, into an exotic Ayurvedic beauty spa.

The word "cosmetic" comes from the Greek *"kosmetikos,"* meaning skill in arranging. The root word, *"kosmos,"* means order. The term perfectly reflects the ancient belief that beauty, indeed, is born of harmonizing your lifestyle as well as bringing order to the mind and inner workings of the body. Ayurvedic cosmetics are one more way, along with Ayurvedic diet and lifestyle practices, to help towards the ends just described.

Using herbs, flowers, essential oils and naturally occurring minerals, Ayurvedic cosmetics bring the skin to its own perfect balance. In a subtle, soothing way they gently allow us to discover our own natural beauty. Just as with all tissues, the skin must be kept exquisitely clean, well nourished, moisturized, and protected from harm in order to both look and feel its best. Cleansing, nourishing, and protecting are the key factors in Ayurvedic skin care.

Whether prepared at home or purchased from a cosmetics company, you will find Ayurvedic cosmetics . . .
• simple, gentle, and natural
• pleasurable and easy to use
• free from chemicals, mineral oils, petroleum-based products or synthetic perfumes
• free from animal by-products that require killing (milk, cream, and ghee are used as well as lanolin from sheep's wool)
• do not use animal testing
• work to bring balance to the totality of the individual body, mind, and spirit.

The introduction of Ayurveda into modern beauty practices is like going "back to the future;" ancient ingredients and age old procedures speeding toward the cutting edge of today's beauty care. More and more experienced beauty therapists acknowledge that natural cosmetics are more healthy and effective than their synthetic counterparts. They also are aware that people today are beginning to demand total natural body care. There is increasing interest in treatments that work not only to beautify the skin but also to nurture and relax the whole of our being. Ayurveda is a leader in this "new wave" of self-care consciousness.

Totally traditional recipes were designed for Indian people living and working in their homeland, using only what was locally grown, available, and/or affordable. Although fully traditional in approach, the recipes offered here embrace ingredients from both east and west. True to Ayurvedic principles, but adapted for people in today's western world, these recipes use the best ingredients from many parts of the world, especially western herbs, flowers, oils and natural minerals. Integrating these into an Ayurvedic approach is a challenge, but I truly believe that it is the way for Ayurveda to find a new home and help care for needs of the west. In a time of fragmented traditions and whole world consciousness, it is my personal hope that Ayurveda, whether for beauty or general health maintenance, will broaden and adapt to include the best from many cultures and thus be able to appropriately care for people of all colors, cultures, and backgrounds.

Although it is always important to take *prakruti*, or constitution, into consideration when selecting appropriate herbs, oils, and other cosmetic ingredients, the emphasis in this chapter is placed on the condition or *vikruti* of a person's skin and selecting the appropriate ingredients that possess the needed qualities and actions to remedy that condition. The qualities and actions emphasized here are whether an ingredient or formula is cleansing, moisturizing, or toning. This being said, always please bear in mind that addressing the condition of the skin alone is a symptomatic approach. Thus you may need to alter what you do to your skin on a day-to-day basis.

Of course, there are always the constants of one's constitution which give the skin certain characteristics. Skin conditions that are exacerbations of your dosha dominance will always take longer to address. But even these conditions, as well as ones that are more acute, are affected by so many other factors such as diet, lifestyle, climate, mental state, and general health. It is for these reasons that it is wise not to be too rigid in addressing your skin and it's condition based solely on constitution. Living in accordance with your constitution and strengthening it will go a long way in bringing out the natural beauty of your skin, but you always need to pay attention to daily needs and addressing the factors that challenge you. Topical treatment together with a positive health-supporting lifestyle are equal partners on the journey toward a vital, glowing complexion.

Earlier it was said that those conditions that are in keeping with one's dosha dominance are more difficult to address than those that are solely the result of aberrant diet and lifestyle which bring out symptoms of another dosha. Here are some practical examples of what I mean . . .

Mrs. Jones has a Vata dominant constitution and has a problem with cracked lips. Dry lips are a reflection of the internal dryness in the lower digestive tract, a situation symptomatic of Vata constitution. Because the condition is in keeping with her constitution, Mrs. Jone's problem is liable to take longer to remedy. As a more deep-seated problem is being indicated by her dry lips, she will need to pay more attention to her full body health in order to restore her constitutional balance and eliminate her cracked lips.

If, however, the condition is not associated with dominant dosha balance, it will be easier to work with, possibly needing only temporary topical care.

Ms. Brown has an itchy red rash on her eye lids. This is a Pitta-type condition, but her constitution is more Vata-Kapha. She observed the rash arising after using a new eye make-up. More than likely this is just an allergic reaction that has made Pitta-dosha flare up locally on the eyelid and will be relatively easily cared for by a soothing creme.

Understanding the nature of the cause of any problem is the real science of Ayurvedic healing. Bringing the body back to balance, by whatever means, is the art. I hope that what is provided below helps you to develop these skills and reap their benefits.

A Refresher on Skin Types Associated with Dosha Dominance

For the sake of convenience, characteristic skin types associated with Vata, Pitta, and Kapha are, again, listed here. I've also mentioned common complaints that arise when a particular dosha is out of balance. These symptoms or conditions are a dosha's vikruti.

Vata Prakruti
- thin, fine pored, darker complexion with a whitish or grayish hue
- cool to the touch, especially in the extremities (hands and feet) and dry or rough and flaky in patches
- climate sensitive

Vata Vikruti
- lack of tone or luster
- rough patches, chapping and cracking
- dry rashes
- corns and callouses
- dry eczema

Pitta Prakruti
- fair, peachy, coppery, or freckled complexion
- soft. lustrous, and warm
- chemically sensitive

Pitta Vikruti
- rashes, inflammation, itching
- oily 'T' zone
- premature wrinkling
- yellow pustular acne, blackheads, whiteheads, general excessive oiliness
- discoloration of natural pigmentation

Kapha Prakruti
- thick, moist, pale
- soft and cool to the touch, generally
- tones well, ages well

Kapha Vikruti

- dull, sluggish, congested skin
- enlarged pores
- blackheads or large white pustules or cystic formations
- thick, oily secretions

Don't worry about integrating all of this material at once. With study, practice, and experience you will better understand Ayurveda and how its techniques interpret and manipulate the phenomenal world. As this understanding develops within you, you will become a master in kosmetikos, bringing beauty and order to your body, then sharing it with those you love, and the whole world around you.

FACIAL TREATMENT

There are eight steps in a full Ayurvedic facial treatment:
1. cleansing
2. oleation massage
3. herbal steam or compress
4. gentle scrub
5. cleansing or nutrifying mask/facial pack
6. toning/rejuvenating
7. moisturizing
8. hydrating
9. application of make-up (optional)

Cleansing, toning, and moisturizing are sufficient on a daily basis. (Steps 1, 6,7) Do the full program once a week or at least twice a month.

Each of the steps are thoroughly explained in the text below, including how to do each procedure and recipes for each skin type.

The recipes offered in this section provide for basic ingredients with suggestions for adapting formulas for particular skin types and personal preferences. Often people have strong attractions or aversions to scents, so I have tried to offer a variety of "flavors". All of the ingredients are available through sources listed in the Source Appendix. In keeping with the spirit of Ayurveda, as the needs of individuals differ, I do not indicate exact proportions. It is best to trust your intuition and test out what proportions of ingredients create the effect you feel is best. However, if you want to use the techniques but are not so interested in making your own cosmetics, there are a number of excellent Ayurvedic cosmetics available from several companies which are also listed in the Source Appendix. Please remember that just because ingredients are pure and natural does not make them hypoallergenic. Whether you make cosmetics at home or purchase them from a commercial company, test these cosmetics on a small area of skin before you spread them all over your face or body. On a daily basis, cleansing, moisturizing, and a little rejuvenative care is all that is usually needed. The complete program is wonderful to do once a week. You'll find that the time you set aside for yourself will pay dividends. You will look and feel more beautiful, have more strength and stamina, greater clarity of mind and basically feel more confidence in dealing with the demands of the day. For women, time taken for this kind of self nurturing, especially on the first day of your period, can make a tremendous difference in menstrual symptoms and will ease the transitioning through menopause.

INITIAL CLEANSING
Sebum, sweat, and accompanying waste products constantly spill out onto the surface of the skin attracting dirt and offering a home to bacteria. Initial cleansing removes this sticky later as well as make-up, leaving the skin's surface fresh and ready to receive a facial massage.

Traditionally, Ayurveda suggests the use of herbal powders called "ubtans" to cleanse the skin. The powders are mixed with various liquids to form a creamy paste. They are then applied like a very fine scrub. If this does not appeal, then use a natural creme or oil base cleanser, but never use soap on your face. Soap, as I've said before, strips the skin of it's protective mantle robbing it of moisturizing oils and interfering with the natural functioning of the pores and temporarily destroying an important barrier to infection. This is even more important to avoid with delicate facial skin. There are a few Ayurvedic soaps available, such as Chandrika, Sandalwood, and Neem. Use them only on the body, and then only occasionally. They are best used for really grimy hands. Generally, when using any soap, use hand or body lotion or oil immediately afterwards to protect the skin until it can once again re-form the mantle (approx. 20 minutes).

HERBAL CLEANSING POWDERS

The following are general and specific herbal cleansing powder recipes. The general recipe can be individually tailored to one's own skin by altering the liquid it is mixed with. The more specific powder formulas have specific liquid bases to fortify their effects. All of these fine herbal powder mixtures improve circulation, sooth, heal, and bring a glow to the complexion.

General formula: contains equal amounts of aloe vera powder, coriander, calamus, comfrey, cumin, elder flowers, fenugreek, lemon peel, licorice, manjistha, nutmeg, tulsi, sandalwood, vertiver, plus fine lentil or chickpea flour or clay. (all hennas are in powder form)

To use this powder for NORMAL skin, mix it with spring water or an herbal tea of your choice.

To benefit DRY skin, add milk powder and water or use milk, fresh cream, or aloe vera juice.

To benefit OILY or BLEMISHED skin, mix with diluted lemon juice or yoghurt.

To help MATURE skin, add a little wheat germ or rosa mosquita oil for gentle nourishment together with spring water or milk.

Specific formulas:

To benefit DRY skin, combine ashwagandha, citrus peel powder, fenugreek, haritaki, lotus seed, rose petal, shatavari, and tulsi with milk powder and water or fresh milk, cream, or aloe vera juice.

To help OILY or BLEMISHED skin, combine amalaki, brahmi, fenugreek, lotus seed, manjistha, neem, white sandalwood with diluted lemon juice or yoghurt.

For MATURE or CONGESTED skin, combine aloe, ashwagandha, bibitaki, citrus peel, haritaki, jasmine, neem, rose, and eucalyptus with a little wheat germ or rosa mosquita oil with spring water or milk.

Oil-based Cleanser

Creams demand help from chemicals to keep them from separating. The following cleanser is free from chemicals and will separate, but only needs a quick shake before use to bring it back to the right consistency.

5 parts base oil (see below)

4 parts aloe vera gel or juice

1 part each of jojoba, avocado, sunflower, almond and Vitamin E oil and glycerine.

Essential oil (single or in combination) of your choice (20 drops per 2 fl. oz. of combined other ingredients.

The following are base and essential oils for the different skin conditions . . .

For NORMAL skin, use almond oil as a base plus the essential oil combination of basil, rosemary, or lemon.

For DRY skin, use sesame oil as your base plus one of the following essential oil combinations:
- rose or sandalwood, plus jasmine and geranium
- cedar, sandalwood, and rose
- sandalwood, geranium, and rose

For OILY skin, use jojoba oil as the base plus one of the following essential oil combinations:
- lemon and cypress
- bergamot, cypress, and juniper

For MATURE skin, try sesame or jojoba oil as your base plus the essential oil combination of lavender, frankincense, and neroli.

For BLEMISHED skin, use jojoba or sunflower oil as the base plus one of the following essential oil combinations:
- lavender and tea tree
- bergamot and lemon

FACIAL MASSAGE

It is hard not to smile from deep inside after an Ayurvedic facial massage. This intricate massage activates deep centers of the brain, reflex points, energy meridians, and facial circulation to totally soothe the body. Tensions in the neck, shoulders, and face are freed and energy is re-balanced from head to toe. Cold pressed seed and nut oils are selected to work with both skin type and constitution. Herbal extracts and essential oils may be added for their additional healing properties and pleasant fragrances.

Although it is wonderful to receive an Ayurvedic Facial Massage, to date there are few trained in this art in the western world. For those interested in such training, the Source Appendix will refer you to places and practitioners to contact. At the same time, the Ayurvedic Facial Massage Sequence described in this book can be done to oneself. Even if one doesn't have the time to follow this sequence, taking the most beneficial oils for your constitution and condition and massaging them in the direction shown in the diagram below will be most beneficial. Although knowing specific points can create a deeper experience, the object here is to get the beneficial oils deep into the tissues, in which case the strokes shown below will be most adequate.

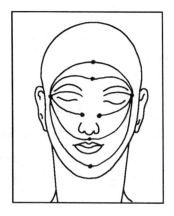

Massage Oils

The basic formula for creating your own individualized massage oil is . . .

10 parts base oil
1 part wheat germ oil
400 IU of Vitamin E oil (usually the equivalent of two capsules) per 6 Tablespoons of wheat germ and base oil
Essential oil combinations; 20 drops per 2 fl. oz. of above combined oils.

The ideal base oil and essential oil combinations to use for various skin conditions are . . .

For NORMAL skin, use jojoba or almond as your base oil and one of the following essential oil combinations:
• lavender, geranium, and rose
• cedar, rose, and jasmine

For DRY skin, use 8 parts of sesame with 2 parts of rice bran oil as your base plus the essential oil combination of rose, geranium, and jasmine.

For OILY skin, use jojoba or sunflower oil as your base plus one of the following essential oil combinations:
• lemon and cypress
• bergamot, cypress, and juniper

For MATURE skin, combine 5 parts jojoba oil, 4 parts calendula oil, and 1 part wheat germ, rice bran, or rosa mosquita oil as your base plus the essential oil combination of lavender, frankincense, and neroli.

For BLEMISHED skin, use jojoba as your base and one of the following essential oil combinations:
• lavender and tea tree
• bergamot and lemon

HERBAL STEAMS

The warmth, moisture, and fragrance of an herbal steam melts away muscular tensions, clears the mind, and lifts the spirit. Steams are one of the oldest traditional ways of deeply cleansing the skin. The moisture softens the dry outer edges of the skin, making them easier to remove, leaving behind a soothed, fresher complexion. The heat boosts facial circulation and activates the pores and glands which brings dirt and body toxins to the surface.

Steams are useful for a number of complexion conditions. They are particularly useful for acned or congested skin for just the reasons given. As well as being a simple and beneficial cleansing process, Ayurveda teaches that applying oil followed by heat helps to balance the Vata dosha. Thus as it is an increase in Vata that brings about all signs of aging, reducing Vata through oleation and steam to the face keeps Vata in check, hence promoting youthful qualities. Wrinkles start to fall away as the face starts to feel fresher, brighter, and really warm.

Frequency of steaming is determined by the condition of your skin. If you have dry or mature skin, steam only once every two weeks. Although steaming is moist, over doing it will actually make the skin drier. Once a week is good for normal or oily skin types.

Herbal Steam Preparation

To make an herbal steam, heat at least 2 pints of spring water to the boil. Add two handfuls of one of the herbal combinations listed below to the water, turn off the heat, cover and allow to steep for about 2 minutes.

Bring the pot to a place where you will be able to comfortably lean over it and relax. Remove the pot lid and add a few drops of essential oil. Have the face about 12 to 18 inches above the liquid's surface, then cover the head and pot with a towel to create a mini steam tent. Five minutes is sufficient; ten minutes is maximum. Some people may find that having their hair covered by a cool terry cloth turban, while over the steam, is more relaxing.

Herbal Steam Ingredients

Every steam needs four types of ingredients: those that increase circulation, those that bring out impurities, those that sooth and heal, and some for the therapeutic quality of their aroma. To accomplish this, there are some herbs that are standard to all of the formulas given below. Bay leaf draws circulation towards the skin's surface. Licorice pulls out impurities. The other herbs mentioned have soothing, healing qualities for the skin. Essential oils enhance the aroma as well as activate brain centers and please the mind and relax the body. Use 10 drops per 2 pints of water.

For NORMAL skin, use a combination of licorice, rose, sandalwood, thyme, ashwagandha, bay leaf, chamomile, clover, comfrey, fennel, lavender, lady's mantle, marshmallow, and rose plus an essential oil of lavender, geranium, bergamot, or sandalwood.

For DRY skin, try a combination of bay leaf, licorice, chamomile, comfrey, dashmula, dandelion, rose, sandalwood, marshmallow, and orange peel. This combination can be used about once a month. However, for dry skin a warm compress is more gentle. Try an herbal tea decoction made from comfrey, elder, lavender, lime flower, rose, rosemary, sandalwood, and yarrow or 3 to 4 drops of essential oil of rose, sandalwood, chamomile, or neroli per 2 pints of boiled spring water. (See more about compresses below.)

For OILY skin, try a combination of bay leaf, licorice, comfrey, fennel, lavender, lemon balm, lemon grass, lemon peel, lemon verbena, rose, rosemary, and sandalwood (or witch hazel bark) with the essential oil combination of juniper, lemon, and cypress.

For MATURE skin, try bay leaf, licorice, anise, cinnamon, clove, eucalyptus, fennel, ginger, mint, nettle, orange peel, and pine with the essential oil of rosemary or sage.

For BLEMISHED skin, use a combination of bay leaf, licorice, blackcurrant leaf, burdock root, dandelion root, lemon grass, manjishta, and yarrow with essential oil of blue chamomile, myrrh, rose, lemon, bergamot, lavender, cedar, or juniper.

More on the Use of Compresses

Compresses are an excellent alternative to a steam. Warm or cool compresses provide many of the benefits of steam without the risk of drying out the skin. Their gentle action swells the outer dry layers of skin and then stimulates the skin activity just like a steam. The skin becomes soft, smooth, and more receptive to further treatment. Compresses are best for very dry, sensitive skin or when the skin is flushed and prone to thread veins. Use 2 pints of liquid (For ingredients, refer to dry skin section for herbal steam), or whatever is sufficient to totally immerse a wash cloth. Wring out the cloth and apply it to the face. Either cut holes for eyes, nose, and mouth or use two cloths; one to cover the eyes, nose, and cheek, the other for the chin and jaw.

SCRUBS

A scrub should be mild and unabrasive enough to be able to be used every day. Scrubs stimulate circulation and cleanse the pores, preventing blackheads by efficiently removing the dead scaly outer most layer of the skin. They bring a glowing luster to the complexion and stimulate new skin growth. Formulated for your skin type, it can be used instead of soap or cleanser on a daily basis or as part of your weekly facial ritual.

Avoid scrubs claimed to be natural that use crushed apricot pits or nut shells as they are too rough and abrasive. (This means that it is also best to avoid using buffing pads and loofas on the facial skin.) The action of such products could be likened to trying to bring a smooth, perfect finish to wood using only rough sand paper. They can also irritate and cause microscopic damage to the fragile structures of the skin.

Generally, the base of all scrubs are whole grain or bean flour with some powdered herbs added for deeper cleansing and powdered dried flower petals for scent and color. Like the ubtans, they are mixed with sufficient spring water or herbal tea to make a creamy paste. (You can use a little of the herb tea or essential oil water from your steam.)

Gently rub the mixture on the face in small, clockwise circles. Rinse off with cool, clean water.

For NORMAL skin, use oat flour plus a little tulsi, sandalwood powder, and powdered rose petals. Mix to a paste with spring water, raw milk, or comfrey tea.

For DRY skin, use chickpea or fine lentil flour with wheat germ, powdered almonds, agar agar, ashwagandha, haritaki, fenugreek, tulsi, elder flowers, and rose petals. Mix these ingredients with aloe vera juice, milk, or cream.

For OILY skin, use barley flour with rice bran, amalaki, coriander, manjishta, neem, sandalwood, and lavender powder. Mix these with dilute lemon or aloe vera juice.

For MATURE skin, use lentil, barley, or rice flour with haritaki, ashwagandha, tulsi, licorice, and powdered orange blossom mixed with aloe vera juice or milk with a little honey.

For BLEMISHED skin, use oat flour and clay powder plus ashwagandha, coriander, cumin, bibitaki, haritaki, fenugreek, ginger, neem, manjishta, and a pinch of turmeric and lavender powder all mixed with yoghurt.

All of these scrubs can be used as masks. What follows are more specific beneficial facial masks.

MASKS
There are many types of masks, but basically their actions fall into three categories: 1) They extract dirt from deep in the skin, preventing or eliminating blackheads and acne. 2) They nourish by providing vitamins and minerals and rejuvenate by refining pores, healing scarring, evening out the color tone, soothing and moisturizing the skin. 3) They can also stimulate the deepest layer of the skin to make healthy new growth.

Clay is the best base for a mask as it acts like a magnet for dirt and toxins that accumulate deep in the skin. Clay is also a rich source of minerals (vital to healthy skin), such as iron, magnesium, zinc, potassium, calcium, and silica. Powdered white or green clay is available in most health food and herb shops.

To make a mask most effective for you, select herbs and essential oils in accordance with your skin condition (viz. selection for steams). Only a few drops of essential oil are needed to create a pleasant fragrance. A mask should be worn for 10 to 20 minutes. Use this time to do a quick hand and foot massage.

For NORMAL and DRY skin, create a mask with 6 parts clay, 2 parts aloe vera juice, egg white, or spring water, and 1 part honey.

For OILY skin, make a mask with 5 parts clay, 1 part honey, 1 part aloe vera juice, and 1 part fennel tea or lemon juice.

For MATURE skin, use 6 parts clay, 3 parts honey, 2 parts spring water or aloe vera juice, plus a little rosa mosquita, Vitamin E and A, evening primrose, or borage oil.

For BLEMISHED skin, try 6 parts clay, 1 part yoghurt, and 2 parts jojoba oil.

FACE PACKS

Face packs are softer and more porous types of face masks. Very similar in action, they improve circulation as well as cleanse and tauten the entire face. Because they are soft, they allow the skin to breathe more and are gentler than masks, they can be left on longer, even during a full body massage.

The face packs discussed here are made of a variety of fruits and vegetables. The juices of fresh fruits and vegetables tone and provide enzymes that help balance and cleanse the skin.

Mash or pulp the fresh fruit and vegetables, then add fruit pectin, agar agar, clay or oat flour to firm the mixture so it does not slide off the face.

For NORMAL skin, use avocado, banana, cantaloupe, grape, peach, nectarine, or zucchini.

For DRY skin, try apple, avocado, banana, carrot, pear, melon, or nectarine.

For OILY skin, use cabbage, cucumber, lemon, pear, strawberry, or tomato.

For MATURE skin, choose apple, avocado, grape, or lemon.

For BLEMISHED skin, try apple, cabbage, grape, or tomato.

Both masks or packs should be removed with cool water and a clean wash cloth.

TONERS

A good toner is a non-alcohol refresher that helps remove the residue of all the previous procedures. It refines the pores and tautens and tones the skin, making it ready for moisturizing treatment.

Aftershave is basically a toner. However, because most aftershaves are primarily made of alcohol and perfume, they damage the skin by disturbing the recovery of the mantle which is destroyed by shaving soap and razor blade. The alcohol will further dry the skin.

Rather than such abrasive products, try using mild astringents or essential oil mists. Apply toner with a cotton ball or spray on with a hand pump mister.

Try one of the following toners, selecting one on the basis of your skin condition.

For NORMAL skin, combine witch hazel with an equal amount of an herbal tea or floral water. Suitable herb teas include comfrey, elder flower, or rosemary. Nothing tops really high quality rose water.

For DRY skin, use pure rose water.

For OILY skin, use tulsi water or a mixture of equal amounts of witch hazel with cilantro, fennel, dead nettle, or yarrow tea.

For MATURE skin, use pure rose water.

For BLEMISHED skin, use equal amounts of witch hazel with either tulsi or rose water.

MOISTURIZERS

All types of skin need moisturizer, even those that are oily by nature. Moisturizers protect the skin from the elements by acting as physical barriers. It also protects the skin from invasion by bacteria and keeps make-up out of the pores.

Moisturizing action is twofold. It plumps up the outer layers of the skin, making it soft, silky, and smooth, temporarily removing tiny wrinkles and disguising deeper ones. It also prevents dry air from "pulling" moisture out of the skin. Glycerine is an ingredient of many moisturizers which works by drawing the skin's moisture to the surface. This is fine, so long as there is sufficient moisture in the body to replace it and keep the deeper layers of the skin well lubricated. If not, the long term effect will be a deep drying and loss of skin tone. Besides glycerine, many moisturizers and body lotions contain alcohol. Alcohol is drying in nature, so it is also not useful in the long run. Try to avoid moisturizers with these products unless you know that your skin has sufficient moisture within.

Moisturizers should be applied after every washing to help replace the skin's mantle (which takes approx. 20 minutes). Lighter moisturizer is best during the day, a heavier, more nourishing one at night when the skin is more receptive to nourishment.

The basic proportions for a moisturizer are:

2 Tablespoons aloe vera gel

3 ounces of oil

1 ounce of cocoa butter or lanolin

2 ounces of rose water

For NORMAL skin, use almond or jojoba oil.

For DRY skin, use sesame oil or lanolin.

For OILY or BLEMISHED skin, use jojoba oil or jojoba butter.

For MATURE skin, use rice bran oil or ghee.

To prepare, warm the oils and butter together and the floral water and aloe vera separately. Place all of the ingredients in a blender and whip. Add essential oils as used for the different massage oils discussed. To make a heavier night cream, decrease the amount of aloe vera gel and add Vitamin E and A or a little rosa mosquita oil. Keep in an air tight jar in a cool place.

The area around the eyes needs special care because the tissues around the eyes have no oil glands. This area is also tender and often sensitive. Avoid pulling on this area when massaging or applying make-up. It is easily stretched. Also avoid applying drying masks to this area. Dab pure rosa mosquita oil around the eyes at night time. This will prevent deepening of wrinkles that will naturally appear over time.

Wrinkles can be viewed in different ways. View them as signs of wisdom, showing a deepening of character. Let them also be laugh lines, evidence of a life full of joy and contentment rather than the fixed scowl of bitterness. Remember, the body never lies—especially the face.

MISTS

The gentle touch of a spray mist brings vitality back to the complexion any time of day. Mists are wonderful in very dry climates, in windy weather, after exercise, or during times of air travel when the skin is particularly susceptible to dehydration. Use them to stabilize make-up, re-activate moisturizer, or just as an uplifting refresher anytime. Apply a mist before and after moisturizing to assist absorption.

Mists may be made of pure spring water, an herbal tea, or water enhanced with minerals. One of the specialties in Ayurveda is using metals, minerals, and gems for healing. The qualities of precious metals can be conveyed to water by boiling the metal with water in a glass or enamel pan. Use 1 ounce of metal per 20 fluid ounces of water, simmering until half of the water is gone. (If you do not have as much as an ounce of a metal, use a heavy ring and place it in 1 pint of water.) This water can then be used as a spray mist.

For NORMAL or DRY skin, use gold water.

For OILY skin, use silver water.

For MATURE skin, use copper or gold water.

For BLEMISHED or CONGESTED skin, use copper water.

A mist using gem water can also be made. The qualities of gems are conveyed to water by allowing a glass of spring water (with the gem stone in it) to sit in strong sunlight for thirty days. Check the section regarding gem therapy for the beneficial qualities of particular gems.

About Make-up . . .

As your general health improves and your body gets more in balance, so will the quality of your skin. Your natural inner strength and natural beauty will start to shine and you will need less adornment.

Use make-up only when necessary, allowing as much time as possible to be in a completely natural state. Use only top quality natural cosmetics just to enhance—not to cover up—your looks.

And remember . . .

> *"Life is a mirror. If you frown at it,*
> *it frowns back. If you smile,*
> *it returns the greeting."* (Thackeray)

Skin Care for the Whole Body

Ayurvedic full body skin care follows the same principles and procedures as for the facial but uses fewer steps as a number of actions are combined in the same step. In this section I have outlined both a system you can do for yourself at home and a slightly more elaborate alternative that requires a professional massage therapist and spa facilities. Both give excellent results.

Caring For Your Skin at Home

• Apply warmed oil that is appropriate to your dosha dominance and skin condition all over your body. Use simple cold-pressed oil or oil that has been enhanced with herbs and/or essential oils as described in the recipe section, p. 177. (see Blends).

• Give yourself a full body massage. The section on self-massage (p. 124) provides step-by-step instructions. This procedure is particularly invigorating. However, the main idea is to simply work the oil into the skin.

• Increase the heat in your body by exercising. Oiling up and then exercising is very useful for Vata-dominant constitutions and in times of high stress. Alternatively, simply warm the skin by relaxing for twenty minutes in the sun. Use this time for skilled relaxation or quiet reflection. At least avoid unharmonious situations for these few minutes.

• Cleanse yourself with an ubtan. (An ubtan is a mixture of flour, herbs, and sometimes oil that cleanses, tones, nutrifies, and moisturizes the skin.) Apply the ubtan just as you would a facial scrub, but going all over the body. (see p. 178 for recipes) The paste tends to flick about, so the cleanest way to apply it is by sitting in the bathtub. For extra comfort, run a couple of inches of warm water first. The water takes the chill off the tub and can be splashed on the body if the ubtan paste gets a bit dry.

• Take a warm herbal or aromatherapy bath to rinse the ubtan off, followed by a quick cool shower. The warm bath opens up the tissues and the quick cool shower sends blood shooting to the skin's surface. Pat dry and take a few quiet moments for yourself.

You'll feel completely relaxed and pleasantly charged with energy. It's a great way to start the day, taking only about thirty-five minutes—with exercise and relaxation exercise included. It's also a wonderful way to completely let go of the stresses of the day so you can enjoy a productive or fun evening—and get a great night's sleep.

Spa-style Ayurvedic Body Care

• Body Massage—The recipient should receive a full body massage using copious amounts of fragrant, warm oil. Ayurvedic massage uses one or sometimes two massage therapists to rhythmically stimulate the subtle energy flows of the body and relax the skin and underlying muscle tissue. The emphasis here is to make the massage a safe, nurturing experience. Many clients have likened it to returning to the womb.

• Herbal Body Steam—While the oil is still on the body, the recipient takes an herbal steam in a steam box. The moisture of steam stimulates circulation towards the skin's surface and opens up the glands and pores so they can drink up the nourishing oil. The oil moisturizes, making the skin full and supple, while being a carrier for the medicinal properties of the herbs and essential oils. Rest time is given after the steam to cool off a little and relax. (A hot bath does very much the same, especially if it is followed by an herbal wrap that allows the body to get warmed through.)

• Ubvartan—This is vigorously rubbing dry herbs or herbal pastes (ubtans) into the skin. As well as cleansing and nourishing the skin, this process tones the muscles and reduces fat by improving the metabolism of the muscles and adipose tissue. It is very invigorating and leaves the skin tingling, soothed and soft.

• Rinse—A cool rinse is needed to remove the powder or paste completely. Gently pat the body dry and discover how smooth, fresh, and supple the skin feels even without lotion. If in a particularly dry climate, apply a little body oil or lotion if necessary.

For a total Ayurvedic beauty experience, take one of the special treatments before the final rinse off:

Shirodhara—allow the furthermost corners of your mind and body to release and relax as a fine stream of warm sesame oil is poured onto the third eye.

With *netra basti*, the eyes are bathed with warm clarified butter to release the inner tensions of the eye sockets, soothe dry wrinkles, and bring a glamorous sparkle to the eyes.

Offer a short facial massage and give nasya (application of nasal drops) to relax and clear the mind and clear away the darkness from beneath the eyes.

Do *karna purana*, pouring warm oil in the ears and allow it to remain for twenty minutes to relieve jaw and neck tensions.

Recipes and Ingredients for Full Body Skin Care

In describing formulas and herbs for Ayurvedic facials, the emphasis is on how they will impact a given condition of the facial skin. This does take into account constitution, but here, it is constitution that is particularly being addressed. This will mean that all of the herbs and oil combinations suitable for the facial procedures are included, but that the formulas that follow, because they address the whole body will have a greater, overall impact.

Oil Blends

In general, when preparing oils and selecting herbs for the various procedures, one should think about the various dosha dominances in the following manner:

When Vata is dominant—think of preparations that are warming, nourishing, and toning (best for dry skin).

When Pitta is dominant—think of preparations that are cooling, cleansing, and soothing (especially for oily and blemished skin).

When Kapha is dominant—think of preparations that are warming, cleansing, and stimulating (best for normal and mature skin).

VATA BLENDS:

Base Oil—sesame or avocado oil enriched with wheat germ or castor oil

Herbs—ashwagandha, brahmi, comfrey, cinnamon, fenugreek, haritaki, tulsi, shatavari

Essential Oils—clary sage, cinnamon, clove, cypress, geranium, jasmine, musk, rose, sandalwood

PITTA BLENDS:

Base Oil—sunflower or safflower enriched with calendula, coconut, or rice bran oil

Herbs—amalaki, chamomile, coriander, jasmine, mahabala, manjishta, sandalwood

Essential Oils—chamomile, gardenia, geranium, honeysuckle, jasmine, lemon grass, melissa, mint, rose, rosewood, sandalwood, vertivert

KAPHA BLENDS:

Base Oil—olive or almond oil enriched with jojoba, rosa mosquita, or Vitamin A oils

Herbs—ashwagandha, bibitaki, fenugreek, haritaki, neem, eucalyptus

Essential Oils—cedar, cinnamon, eucalyptus, frankincense, musk, patchouli, sage

For Body Steams, follow the instructions for facial steams as found on p. 166. For Baths, check the Lifestyle chapter on p. 83.

Ubtans

The simplest ubtans use flour, oil, and a little turmeric.
An example is . . .

    2 ounces chickpea flour
    1/4 ounce of mustard seed oil
    1/2 teaspoon turmeric powder
    Sufficient liquid to form a paste

Chickpea flour is the most nourishing of flours while mustard oil improves circulation.

To make ubtans that are more dosha appropriate, try the following:

For Vata—oat or lentil flour with avocado or sesame oil, wheat germ or castor oil and milk.

For Pitta—barley or rice flour with safflower or sunflower oil and aloe vera or lemon juice.

For Kapha—corn, blue corn or millet flour with olive, almond, or jojoba oil and spring water.

For extra smoothness and to create a nice sheen all over the body, add a tablespoon of fenugreek powder to the recipes.

Ubtans can also be prepared with just herbal powders. A simple formula that tones all skin types and is made of ingredients readily available in the west is a combination of equal amounts of ashwagandha, dashmula, and licorice powders. Just add a little spring water and rub into the body.

More and more Ayurvedic oil and herbal preparations are being produced and made available commercially. Please find the names and addresses of Ayurvedic product distributors and cosmetic companies in the Source Appendix. When you write or call, be sure to ask for full product and ordering information, as well as product and sample price lists.

AYURVEDIC REJUVENATION THERAPY

Ayurveda is more than a system of natural healing. It is both a science and an art of appropriate living which supports longevity and maximizes human potential. From previous chapters it is clear that Ayurveda offers clear and specific guidance for every individual in the proper choice of diet, living habits and exercise to restore and maintain the body, personality, and higher aspirations of the human spirit. By such means Ayurveda aims to prevent disease and promote natural, radiant beauty and positive health.

Both health promotion and healing are based on the principle that the physical form, internal functionings, and psycho-spiritual make-up of an individual is determined by the doshas: Vata, Pitta, and Kapha, all of which are natural forces having distinct qualities and functions. The body is viewed as a product of these forces that have condensed from the outer environment. Though existing as what seems to be a separate form from the point of birth, the individual remains energetically connected to the world that gave it being throughout its entire life. Interaction between the individual and the environment happens through the interplay of the bodily doshas and the energetic qualities of the given environment. Inappropriate diet, personal habits, lifestyles, repressed emotions, climatic and seasonal factors, along with various other forms of stress, contribute to the disruption of the delicate internal balance of the doshas. Disruption of these subtle forces directly affects agni, interfering with digestion, assimilation, and elimination of food substances and disrupts the natural expression of emotions. When agni is weakened, indigestion and confusion result. Incomplete digestion makes even the purest, most nutritious food the source of toxic material known as *ama*. Once formed, ama then enters the bloodstream, clogging the channels and accumulating in sites where energy is lowest and the body thus most vulnerable. It clouds the mind, making the individual less likely to make choices that support health and beauty.

In Ayurveda, health promotion, beauty management and healing rely on freeing the body of ama, restoring sound cellular nutrition, facilitating complete elimination and re-establishing balance to the doshas. This can gradually be achieved through following appropriate diet and lifestyle and improving agni as previously described. But with modern living being so inherently chaotic, such changes are quite challenging, needing considerable discipline and patience. A faster and deeper cleansing and re-balancing can be accomplished through using Ayurveda's traditional rejuvenation therapy.

Commonly called *Pancha Karma*, Ayurvedic rejuvenation therapy is the oldest scientific system for detoxification and re-nutrifying the body in the world today. Although from ancient times it is commonly regarded as one of the most thorough systems available, achieving transformative results on all levels. It rejuvenates the whole system, bringing youthfulness and strength to the body and calm openness to the mind. The combination of oleation massage, full body steam, and flour scrub beautifies the skin making it soft, smooth, and well-toned. While the specific cleansing therapies and rejuvenative tonics work on the internal body, they strengthen the foundations of outer beauty and promote strength of character.

Ayurvedic Rejuvenation Therapy can either be used as a program to improve good health, enhance natural good looks, or initiate the cure of a disorder. Traditionally undertaken as a preventive therapy at the change of seasons, both winter to spring and summer to fall, the aim is to cleanse the body not only of waste materials that may have built up in the body, but also excesses in subtle energies or doshas, thereby promoting positive health and longevity, and balanced beauty through the changing climatic conditions. Traditional analogies describe how it is better to clean the cloth before proceeding with the dying process or to wash a bowl before using it for tea. The meaning here is that in cleansing the body before giving healing foods or herbal medicine will bring a better result.

Rejuvenative therapy should never be considered a replacement for appropriate diet and lifestyle just as an annual vacation should not be the only means to deal with job related stress. Rejuvenation therapy should be viewed as an integral part of on-going self care that helps beauty be with you throughout life. It is also an excellent, completely fresh start in the process of making health-supporting lifestyle changes.

As a seasonal "cure," disorders are prevented or treated by first taking away the underlying causes of disease, namely the toxic wastes that block normal functioning of the body and doshic balance, and then nourishing effected tissues. As a primary healing therapy, thorough cleansing of the body makes it more receptive to medications and tonics as well as increasing the body's ability to fully metabolize foods. Thus, not only are the causes and symptoms of a disease removed, but the body is strengthened—preventing disorders in the future. If you are in good health, Ayurvedic Rejuvenation Therapy will even bring disorders that have not yet manifested symptoms to balance.

It is important to note that once the Pancha Karma process has been completed, the channels of the body are so deeply cleansed and free flowing and the mind more genuinely open that, diet and lifestyle become more important than prior to rejuvenation therapy. Just as herbal medications are now able to penetrate to the deepest part of the tissues and better habit patterns have space to germinate in the mind, toxins from improper diet and poor mental habits are just as free to penetrate and become locked into the system.

Ayurvedic Rejuvenative Therapy is divided into three main areas of treatment: purva karma, pancha karma, and administration of tonics and rejuvenatives. In all cases a simple diet of grains, mung beans, steamed vegetables, and cooked fruits is advised for a week before the rejuvenation program. No meat, alcohol, refined sugar, yeasted bread, or caffeine should be taken. Such a diet then is continued throughout the treatment period. Fasting is not recommended as the therapy is quite demanding of energy.

Purva Karma

Purva Karma is necessary before applying the Pancha Karma procedures. Purva Karma involves warm oleation massages and application of heat to the body. The aim of this treatment is to mobilize wastes and excess doshas from the tissues and to move them towards the large, hollow organs of the body from which they can be removed by the Pancha Karma processes. The massage is luxurious and deeply relaxing. Either one or two massage therapists work to anoint the body with warm oil and then somewhat vigorously massage it into the skin. Warmth from the oil as well as warmth generated by the friction of massage drives the oil through the skin and into the tissue below. This lubricates both the skin and the deeper tissues, loosening blockages and toxins, toning the muscles, and bringing a radiant glaze to the skin.

Usually sesame oil is used because of its ability to penetrate the skin. If Pitta is unusually high, sesame oil can sometimes cause itching or rashes. In this case, cooling herbs can be added to the sesame oil or jojoba or sunflower oil can be used instead. Other herbal oils may be used to either cleanse or nutrify the skin, support various internal organs, or work to balance the doshas. Medicinal quality essential oils may also be added for these purposes. Check the Massage Oil recipes and methods of preparation and Skin Care section for suggested ingredients. Also, several companies now offer Vata, Pitta, and Kapha balancing oils, using herbal extracts and essential oils. They are light with exotic fragrances that please the body and mind, profoundly enhancing the massage process. A number of traditional herbal oils are also commonly available. There are hundreds of herbal oil blends used for purva karma in India. It is an art and science in itself to be able to prepare and apply them for individual needs. At the same time, excellent results are possible with the simple ingredients and more common oils available here in the West when the Ayurvedic practitioner matches them to one's specific needs.

After nurturing the body with warm oil massage, heat is applied to open the circulatory channels of the body, induce sweating, and allow the oil to penetrate more deeply. Heat is applied to the body in various ways:

• *baspa sweda*—steam bath, usually containing herbs to improve circulation and induce sweating (Bay, eucalyptus, and ginger are commonly used. Others may be used for more specific action.)

• *nadi sweda*—steam heat that is applied to specific points or joints through a heat resistant hose

• *upanaha sweda*—poultices and hot compresses on specific areas

• *tapa sweda*—exposure to dry heat near a fire, sunbathing, in a sauna, or sweat lodge

• *drava sweda*—bathing in a hot herbal bath

• *avagana sweda*—herbal sitz bath

• *padavagaha*—hot herbal foot bath

• *hastavagaha*—hot herbal hand bath

• *dhara sweda*—hot shower on the back

• *unagni sweda*—using applications that are not hot in themselves, but produce heat such as mustard oil, ginger compress, or tiger balm. (In all such processes the head is kept cool by being wrapped in a cold, wet towel or having cool water poured over it so the experience is pleasant and dizziness is avoided.)

These techniques can be seen in many folk medicine systems. For example, when I visited Finland, although I was familiar with the sauna, I did not know that herbs were used in saunas for their specific healing properties. Similarly, purifying herbs are sprinkled on hot rocks in a Native American sweat lodge. Ginger compresses are commonly used in Japan and China for a variety of disorders, both structural and organic. In England, a mustard foot bath is still used by many families to ease the symptoms of a head cold. Working with nature in this way is part of the human heritage of many cultures. Ayurveda stands out in this context as it is one of the most ancient, yet comprehensive systems practiced today.

Steam Baths

Of all the techniques mentioned to bring heat into the body, steam bath is the most widely used method in purva karma. The body is enclosed in a steam box or tent with only the head left exposed. Both the head (and for men, the genitals) are kept cool by having cold water applied on a wet towel. The heating and cleansing effect of the steam is enhanced by the addition of herbs. Equal amounts of ginger root slices, eucalyptus, and bay leaf are commonly used. Once again, there are many combinations specific to individual conditions.

After the steam, there is a period to rest and cool down a little. Once body temperature has normalized, a dusting of warmed chickpea flour/powder is applied to remove the oil that has not been absorbed. This oil cannot be used by the body and contains toxins from the sweating process. If it is allowed to remain on and just underneath the skin surface, it will eventually get re-absorbed by the body, causing indigestion, heaviness, lethargy, and constipation.

Purva karma is done five, seven, or ten days, sometimes a little longer if the healing of a long-term problem is being attempted. Oily skin, hair, and bowel movements show that the process is complete and oil has thoroughly penetrated the body. Just as a pre-greased bowl readily empties out a sticky batter, so a well-oiled body easily lets go of accumulated sticky wastes. The cleansing methods involved in the pancha karma methods that accompany purva karma may, in themselves, sound cathartic. However, with the correct preparation, through having done quality purva karma, they are gently, fully, and comfortably accomplished.

Pancha Karma

To fully nourish the body and mind (*santarpana*) and keep balance in the body's energetic system, the channels (*srotas*) that deliver nutrients and take away wastes must be cleaned and well toned (*apatarpana*). Once these are cleared from the largest channels of the digestive and respiratory tract down to the tiniest capillaries, the tissues will continue to cleanse themselves naturally and become more receptive to both nutrients and medicines. The body can then naturally take care of itself and manifest the beauty nature intended. Also, agni will be improved, thus ensuring that all nutrients are thoroughly ingested and absorbed to nourish the tissues, resulting in less wastes produced. This type of cleansing thus initiates rejuvenation of the whole body, improving the quality of health and removing the signs of aging. The body becomes vital, the mind satisfied, and the doshas flow correctly, maintaining positive health and balance. This balance is the root of lasting beauty.

This deep cleansing of the body of impurities and renutrifying of tissues is traditionally accomplished in Ayurveda by a process called Pancha Karma. Literally, Pancha Karma means "five cleansing actions." Prior to these cleansing actions the body must be prepared through the purva karma processes previously discussed. The five cleansing actions of Pancha Karma are:

Virechana—purgation using laxatives to clear impurities from the small intestine and excesses in Pitta dosha

Bastis (classified as Niruna and Anuvasana)—herbal and/or oily decoction enemas to cleanse and establish the correct functioning of the large intestine and excesses in Vata dosha

Vamana—emetics or induced vomiting to clear impurities from the stomach and excesses in Kapha dosha

Nasya—nasal drops to clear impurities from the head

Rakta Moksha—blood letting or blood purification using herbs. (Although classically considered the fifth of the five actions, it is sometimes omitted and the two forms of bastis are classified separately to make up the number of actions to five.)

After completing the appropriate cleansing procedure, care should be taken to not over tax the digestive system and to protect agni. Drink when thirsty and gradually begin to eat when you feel hunger arise, increasing the complexity of foods over a number of meal times as your system allows. Start with warm water, then go to basmati rice gruel, soft cooked basmati rice, then to split mung beans. After these four meals, go to regular kichadi and then kichadi and steamed vegetables. After these simple meals, one should stick with a diet that is suited to your constitution, but again, simple meals at first.

Rejuvenative Tonics

Once blockages have been cleared and toxins removed from the tissues, driven to the large hollow organs and finally flushed from the system, the body is clean and clear to receive either tonics or medications. These may be in the form of herbal tonics taken orally, nutritive enemas, nourishing nasal drops, or body lotions. Because the system is clean it works very efficiently making all such rejuvenative or healing treatments more thoroughly assimilated, thus quickly effective. An in-depth explanation of the principles and practices of rejuvenative therapy is to be found in Dr. Sunil Joshi's forthcoming work with Lotus Press. This work reflects Dr. Joshi's fifteen years of clinical experience helping thousands of people in his native India and in the West. I am indebted to Dr. Joshi for his inspiration and instruction in this specialized area of Ayurveda. He is indeed a master of this science, getting nothing short of miraculous results.

If you would like to get a small taste of the potential of this approach, try the following routine. Choose a time when you are free from a lot of distractions and concerns, where you can rest and relax. Spring or autumn are the best times of year, so long as the weather is mild.
• Follow a simple diet of Kichadi (a mixture of white basmati rice, split mung beans, and spices—recipes can be found in the information about fasting, p. 63, steamed vegetables, and herbal tea. Take a teaspoon of ghee each morning to help improve agni.

• Each day, take a full body massage with warm sesame oil. You can do this for yourself by following the self-massage sequence provided in this book or receive a massage from a friend or partner.
• Exercise to increase body temperature.
• Remove the excess oil by rubbing the body with warm chickpea flour as described on p. 131.
• Rinse off in a warm shower with a last minute rush of cold water. Pat yourself dry.
• Relax for twenty minutes.
• Follow an intestinal cleansing program available from natural food stores and herbalists. There are several excellent regimens and it is best to talk with local therapists who have experience with brands available in your area.
• Start a program of taking an Ayurvedic tonic, like Chywanprash.

For professional help, guidance, and opportunities to experience full Purva and Pancha Karma treatment, contact one of the Ayurvedic centers or therapists listed in the Source Appendix.

Rejuvenative Procedures and Skin Care

I have used the principles of rejuvenation therapy in designing the Ayurvedic Skin Care Program.

The skin is given an initial light cleansing followed by the purva karma procedures of oleation massage and herbal steam. Purva karma prepares the skin for the deeper cleansing of the pancha karma-type procedures using a flour scrub and cleansing mask. Once the skin is exquisitely clean, it is fresh and open to receive rejuvenative treatment using toners, moisturizers, or hydrating spray mists. Similar procedures can be followed for the entire body which would involve full-body massage, herbal steam in a steam box or sauna, herbal body scrub, followed by body lotion. Recipes are in the skin care section.

As well as these adapted procedures, rejuvenation therapy can be used for a variety of beauty problems. As Ayurveda treats the individual not just a condition, the procedures are specific to the totality of the individual's problems. Thus generic answers are not given here.

Virechana, the use of a laxative relieves conditions caused by a Pitta imbalance such as rashes, itching, oiliness, and yellow inflamed pimples. It will also help calm heated emotions such as anger and irritability.

Bastis are used for Vata imbalances usually associated with dry skin, hair, and nails as well as for re-establishing a more steady, comfortable digestion resolving problems with gas and bloating. Emotionally, this works to help flush out deep seated fears and anxieties.

Vamana is used to clear Kapha-genic symptoms caused by various kinds of congestion such as heavy mucous in the head and upper chest, or water retention, congested skin, and excessive weight. Vamana is also extremely helpful in cleansing emotional problems associated with over attachment and weight problems.

Nasya or nasal applications are described fully in the special treatments chapter because they have such a direct effect on appearance. Nasya opens the face and brings a shine to the eyes. It alleviates dark rings under the eyes while calming and clearing the mind.

Rakta Moksha is rarely used except in the less cathartic form of using blood cleansers. Because the blood quality so immediately impacts the condition of the skin, herbal blood purifiers are used to help resolve complaints associated with allergies and/or other toxic conditions. Such herbs work both on the blood and liver to clear the body of ama, and thus restore the skin to natural beauty. Such herbs include burdock, dandelion, yellow dock, red clover, aloe vera, and manjistha. They can be taken as teas or in combinations in capsule form. Once again, consultation with an Ayurvedic physician is suggested for specific instructions that will ensure the best and safest result.

AYURVEDIC FACIAL MASSAGE

This massage sequence draws on the ancient wisdom of the Tibetan and Indian Ayurvedic systems. Traditionally in these systems, polarity, acupressure, and Swedish-style oleation massage were integrated. In fact, it is only in more recent times that these styles have become separate specialties.

The massage works locally and reflexively: locally to improve the skin and uplift the face, and reflexively to relax and deeply nourish the whole body. The Ayurvedic Facial Massage Sequences are part of a complete beauty treatment which includes herbal steams, scrubs, masks, and moisturizers, but may be given alone with excellent results.

WHAT ARE THE BENEFITS OF
THE AYURVEDIC FACIAL MASSAGE SEQUENCE?

• Enhances nourishment and cleansing of tissues which makes for a glowing complexion
• Maintains good tone and elasticity to all skin layers which helps to hold youthful contours
• Melts away facial tension and bodily stress, smoothing wrinkles and brings gentleness to the expression.
• Re-directs subtle energies relieving stiffness throughout the entire body
• Deeply nourishes and strengthens the entire body
• Gives rise to a sensual feeling of joyful excitement that re-energizes the whole body
• Develops a depth of being nurtured that strengthens and increases a willingness to care for others; develops inner beauty

THOUGHTS ON MASSAGE: MAKING CONTACT

Massage means interaction. Wherever we touch the body, change will occur. Not only will it affect the particular site touched, but there will also be a response throughout the entire body. This is commonly recognised in Reflexology where points on the feet, hands, or ears are massaged to help the cleansing and re-energizing of organs, joints, or limbs. It is also recognized in Shiatsu, massage that utilizes acupuncture points to elicit a response in the electromagnetic energy field of the body. In Polarity therapy, this reflexive response is in the subtle fields of energy that surround the body—even the thought forms become unbound from their fixation to the physical body. The Ayurvedic Facial Massage Sequence employs all of these techniques plus oleation massage, concentrating on areas of the face, scalp, neck, and shoulders—commonly tense areas.

Interestingly, if most westerners were asked, "where do you think?" they would point to their heads. Easterners, in contrast, point to their heart region—the center of emotion. This perceptual difference, together with western culture's speed and complexitiy with modern technological lifestyles, creates a focus of a lot more energy in the upper regions of the body (i.e. head, neck, shoulders). Thus, in this modern world, our heads tend to feel busier than the rest of our bodies. Our thoughts and emotions tend to constrict and twist the muscles of the face, head, neck, and shoulders particularly. Sometimes we are more aware of one area than another: maybe pain or tension around our eyes, jaw, chest, back of the neck, or one shoulder. This type of discomfort is the way our bodies have of communicating messages to us, letting us know that all is not fine and flowing freely. Releasing the discomfort not only eases the pain in these areas, but may also release memories, emotional traumas, and/or visual images. Releasing neck tension, for example, allows energy to flow more freely between the head and the heart. This facilitates better connection between our thoughts and emotions, our habits and patterns. The shoulders are often tight due to unexpressed or repressed feelings, as is the jaw. When this tension is released, communication flows more naturally with more confidence and less anxiety.

By working on the head, neck, and shoulders many changes can be facilitated. With such potential, it is very important to work with concentrated care and gentleness. Keep in touch with the other person throughout the session and help them to keep in touch with themselves. If anything of a serious nature comes up, suggest further professional guidance, although it is my observation that Ayurvedic treatments are self-resolving in that many times disturbing feelings come to light, are noted, then leave, never causing problems again. Just as adding Indian spices to your food improves digestion, adding these techniques to your regime of regular self-care can help improve mental digestion, leaving nothing undealt with or haunting.

Throughout the massage description, I have chosen to use the word "friend" for the person receiving massage. They may be your relative, client, lover. Whoever they are, they should be treated with your greatest kindness and respect in true friendship. So the word "friend" is there to remind you of this as you flick through the instructions.

OILS FOR FACIAL MASSAGE

Oil is excellent for the skin, providing it with needed nutrients, lubrication, and protection. It is also the ideal carrier for herbal compounds and essential oils.

Select the base oil according to constitution and condition.

For VATA or dry skin, use sesame, avocado oil or ghee.

For PITTA or oily skin, use sunflower, safflower, or coconut oil.

For KAPHA or moist, sluggish skin, use almond or olive oil.

Jojoba oil is good for all skin types. It is absorbed quickly, leaving very little residue. Its one drawback is that it is the most expensive.

To enrich the base oil, for every 10 parts of base oil add 1 part of Wheat Germ or Vitamin E oil. Add a little rosa mosquita or carrot seed oil for skin that is scarred, extra dry, or needs healing. Essential oils can also be added for their wonderful therapeutic effects and marvellous fragrances. They deepen the pleasure of the massage experience. Select them according to constitution and condition. Use 20 drops per 2 fl. ounces of base oil.

For Vata or dry skin, select the following mixtures:
- sandalwood, geranium, ylang ylang, rosewood
- rose, jasmine, geranium
- cedarwood, sandalwood, rosewood

For Pitta or oily skin, select the following mixtures:
- lemon, cypress
- bergamot, orange, geranium
- cypress, juniper

For Kapha or mature skin, select the following mixtures:
- lavendar, frankincense or myrrh, neroli,
- patchouli, frankincense
- geranium, jasmine

If inflammation is present, select mixtures of:
- roman chamomile, lavendar
- sandalwood, cedarwood,
- rosewood, neroli, rose

If the skin is very wrinkled, select the following mixtures:
- fennel, lavendar, rose,
- frankincense, cypress

If there is deep acne, select one of the following mixtures:
- bergamot, juniper, cypress,
- tea tree, lavendar

For more details, check the aromatherapy portion of this book. Use only medicinal quality essential oils. Always dilute them in proportions suggested and skin test for sensitivity. Aromatherapy is becoming very popular now. With this popularity, the quality of aromatherapy oils has become quite varied. I suggest you use reputable mail order services as suggested in the Source Appendix found at the end of this book.

PREPARING YOURSELF TO GIVE MASSAGE

When massaging someone else, you must remember that everything you are thinking and feeling will be communicated to the person you are working with through simply touching of your fingers to their skin. To make the massage of greatest benefit it is important to try and keep your thoughts pure and your intentions always for the highest good. To help you do this, take a few minutes for yourself before any massage work to calm your body and clear your mind.

Start by sitting comfortably with your back straight. Tuck the chin in a little to release strain in your neck. Place your tongue just behind your front teeth and gently breathe in and out. Let your mind follow the outward breath and naturally relax as you inhale. Bend the elbows, bringing your hands to the level of your heart. Let your shoulders melt and drop towards the floor. Relax your hands to form a gentle cup shape. Imagine your hands are being filled with intense light condensing from the heavens. Allow the light to flow through your hands, elbows, and shoulders, then towards your heart in a clear stream. Feel the light filling your heart and accept the strength and joy it brings. Let this sensation fill your whole body. Rest in that space, letting your mind notice each and every part of your body and all your thoughts and feelings.

When you are ready, rub the backs of your hands vigorously, then rub your palms together for a few moments. Cup your hands in front of you, yet not touching—as if holding a ball and feel the energy between your fingers. Direct your mind to the benefit of your friend, remembering it is not you, but the clear energy of the universe working through you that really does the work. Apply warm oil to your hands and when your friend is ready, begin.

Along with this clear and positive mental state of mind, you will do your best work when you feel balanced both mentally and physically, so take time to take care of yourself. At the same time, massage is a two-way business. In the process of engaging the recipient of your massage, encourage them to feel physically comfortable and be open, trusting in your work.

After the massage, both giver and the receiver should rest for a brief period to once again gather and balance the energy in both of your bodies. For the giver, a high energy snack of warm milk, nuts, dates, and raisins may also be taken to ensure that there is no overall loss of vital energy.

Allow your intuition to guide the rhythm and pressure of the massage. Focus on staying relaxed. Individual constitutional types will generally prefer and benefit from different styles of treatment.

Vata people enjoy subtle energy work: light touch, warmth, and gentleness. When talking to them, be soft, supportive and use feeling tones and music. (A sample dialogue for Vata types using imagery . . . "Allow yourself to float back and enjoy the warmth and aroma of the oil. Let it caress your face and melt away your tensions, taking you to a quiet, still, creative space within.")

Pitta people enjoy direct, firm, cool and refreshing touch. They also enjoy logical explanations of the work and color-visual imagery. (A sample dialogue for Pitta types using imagery . . . "Lay back. Notice each point where your body touches the table. Allow a cool blue light to pass through you, relieving your tensions and transporting you to a place among loving friends, filled with soft colors and luxurious sensations.")

Kapha people benefit most from firm, deeply stimulating touch. They need to be motivated to keep in touch with the massage process rather than drift into sleep. Any insights you share with them will go deep and be long lasting. (A sample dialogue for Kapha types using imagery . . . "Allow my touch to gradually penetrate deep into your tissues bringing with it a sense of light, fresh, tingling, dancing energy to awaken and inspire your deepest thoughts and sensations.")

PRELIMINARY MASSAGE PROCEDURES

The most pleasant and effective way to begin a session of beauty massage is to work briefly on the spine. Using tapping, rubbing, firm pressure, and herbal compresses, the spine can be gently urged to relax and resume its natural shape. Correct alignment and strength of the spine gives the whole body gentle grace, poise, and confident command. A strictly physical spinal massage strengthens the nervous system and promotes the flow of cerebral-spinal fluid. This helps with emotional balance. On a more subtle level it allows the life giving energies of the body to flow freely which keeps the body vital, youthful, and glamorous longer than would normally be expected.

For the massage, the receiver needs to be lying on their front with their back exposed from the sacrum up to the top of the neck. Always make your massage strokes so that they start from the base and work up to the top of the spine.

Start by tapping in a bouncy action using a "hacking" action whereby the hands are stretched out and the fingers loosely spaced. This awakens the spinal energies and improves circulation to the spinal area.

Next take warm oil and vigorously rub it into either side of the sacrum, then up along both sides of the vertebral column. Generally sesame oil is good because it penetrates well, lubricating the connective tissues of the spine. If there is stiffness or misalignment, use Mahanarayan or mustard oil, or equal parts of ginger juice and sesame oil. Rub vigorously to get the oil absorbed. Then using both thumbs, apply pressure evenly, starting at the tip of the sacral area, then on both sides of the sacrum and up the spine. Pressure should be firm, but not uncomfortable. If pressure is too strong you will see the body physically brace in anticipation of the next pressure point.

Finally, apply a hot ginger compress over the sacral area (use ginger tea recipe found on p. 51 and saturate a folded wash cloth with this tea). Let the heat penetrate and when the compress is cool, remove, dip in the hot tea, and reapply. Do this for a total of three times until the skin is noticeably pink. Dry the sacral area and wipe off the excess oil from the spine with the hot (ginger saturated) cloth.

Have the recipient turn over, then slip a hot pad under their sacral area to keep it warm. Do not use an electric heating pad as it disturbs the subtle energies of the body. A hot water bottle or chemical hot/cold pack is best (both are available at most pharmacies). If you are not able to take the time or do not have a suitable set-up to follow the entire spinal procedure as described here, at least place the hot pad on the sacrum. It helps the neck and shoulder muscles release and relax tremendously. If the recipient is cold or nervous, use a hot pad just below the navel on the lower abdomen. This can also help with headaches caused by deep abdominal tension.

Step One
Standing or kneeling behind your friend, cradle the back of their head in your cupped hands. Close their ear holes with your thumbs and place your finger tips along the ridge of the skull at the back of the head. Feel the weight of their head in your hands. The more relaxed

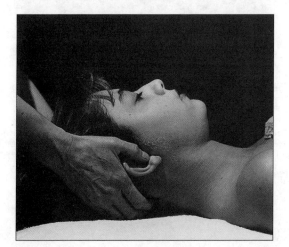

the person is, the heavier their head will feel in your hands. Note that the more you relax your own arms, you will assist them in letting go more easily.

Ask your friend to "let go" and allow you to do the moving as you bring their chin forward to their chest, stretching the curve of their neck, holding their head in this position to the count of three. If there is pain or stiffness rock the head gently between your two hands. Then allow the head to rest on the table for a few moments. Repeat this process two more times; raising, then gently lowering the head. (Sometimes during the treatment, the neck tightens again. You will notice this by the chin pointing more in the air than being in a slightly tucked position. If you see this, re-adjust the head, using this gentle stretch technique.)

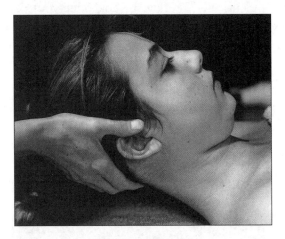

Step One establishes a non-invasive contact with the person, building rapport and mutual confidence.

BENEFIT: Releasing neck tension which initiates a "relaxation" response in the whole body by opening up the flow of energy from the spine into the whole head.

Step Two

Keep the head cradled in your hands, moving only your thumbs to be in front of the ears. Breathe in as your friend breathes out and out as your friend breathes in. Center yourself by breathing down into your *Hara,* a point two to three inches below your navel. Send out positive thoughts. This is called "touching the subconscious." It creates a deeper contact with the person, harmonizing your energies. You may also use verbal suggestions at this point.

"Allow each breath to nourish and relax your body. Let those feelings build until they are all you perceive. Each breath makes your body more relaxed, yet vital, and your mind more peaceful, yet clear. Each breath charges your sense organs, bringing joy into your life."

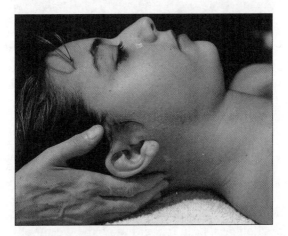

Again, remember that the more present and relaxed you are, the easier it is for your friend to relax. If at any point you feel that you have lost your focus or contact, return to this breathing pattern.

BENEFIT: Balances the electromagnetic energies in the right and left side of the brain. This reduces stress as it increases the brain's ability to deal with incoming information, bringing both the logical and intuitive responses together.

Step Three

Change your hand position so that the left hand is cradling the back of the head and the right hand wraps over the forehead. Use the same alternate breathing as in Step Two for about 90-120 seconds.

BENEFIT: Balances the electromagnetic energies of the front and the back of the brain. This can help bring forward deeply buried memories to the conscious mind and release them.

Steps Two and Three help to create an alert, balanced state of calm and receptivity.

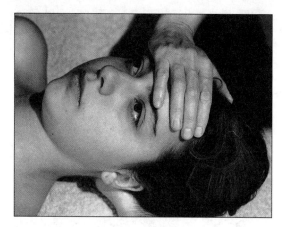

Step Four

Rest the heels of your hands midway between the neck and the tips of the shoulders. Lean forward using the weight of your body to push the shoulders down towards the toes. (This is less tiring than using only the strength of your arm muscles.) Repeat once or twice.

BENEFITS: After holding a stretched posture, the muscles of the shoulders naturally relax, balancing the position of the shoulder girdle. As the shoulders relax the pelvic girdle responds by adjusting slightly as well. When the two girdles release their tension, energy can flow more freely between them throughout the torso. Breathing will become deeper and easier. Sometimes the person receiving the massage

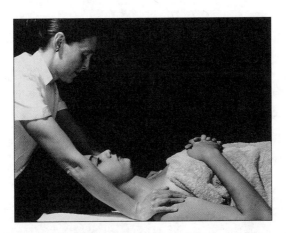

will sigh or take a very long, visible deep breath. This type of breath is a good sign of deep release.

Step Five

Move to the right side of your friend at the level of their knees. Rest your left hand on the large thigh muscle on the front of the right leg and cup the right knee cap in the palm of your right hand. Rotate the knee cap five times counter-clockwise and five times clockwise. Counter-clockwise movements are more stimulating and clockwise

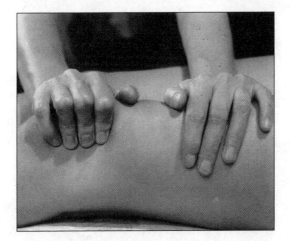

movements are more calming. So first we stimulate, then calm the energy. Remaining on your friend's right side, reach over to the left leg and repeat the same procedure.

Keeping both hands in contact with your friend is more balancing and re-assuring. Try to do this for each move, even when only one hand is active.

BENEFIT: Releases hidden tension that accumulates around the knees. This is most common among people who have to stand for long hours.

Step Six

Move to your friend's feet and stand so that you are looking straight up the body. Make a "V" shape between your thumb and fingers. Slide your hands up the lower legs over the shins until they are just below the knees. You will feel the large bone ends just before the knee joint on the inner side of the knee. Allow your thumbs to rest just below where these bones end. As in Step Four, apply a light pressure to these points, leaning toward the person so that the emphasis of the pressure is towards the hips. Do not press down toward the table as this could damage the knees. Massage the point under your thumbs in small clockwise circles.

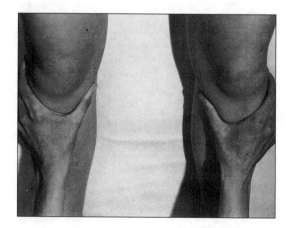

BENEFITS: Balanced energy is gradually brought down from the head, neck, and shoulders to the legs. The point to the inside of the knees helps build strength and stamina. It is particularly useful for those who have been under long term stress, i.e. if they have things in their lives they cannot stand. Also useful to give extra energy for long car or plane journeys.

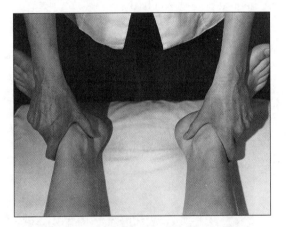

Step Seven

Move the hands down towards the ankles. Rest the thumbs at the point midway between where the back of the heel touches the ground and the bone which protrudes on the inner side of the ankle. These are the negative pole points of the body as the head is the positive pole. Apply gentle pressure and lean forward again two or three times, the emphasis of the lean being towards the hips.

BENEFIT: Touching first the head or body's positive pole and working down to the ankles or the negative pole while focusing on the breath, moves and balances the body's electromagnetic flow, harmonizing and relaxing the body.

Step Eight

Move back to your friend's right side at the level of the chest. Rest your left hand over the forehead and the right hand on the belly, three to four finger widths below the navel. Rub the belly in a clockwise direction slowly five times, then rock the belly by moving your right hand across and back, up and down along the whole abdomen. The belly is the neutral pole of the body.

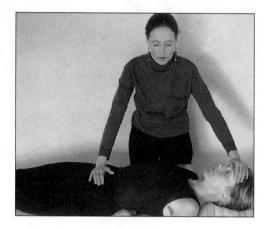

BENEFITS: Much anxiety and tension is held in the muscles of the abdomen and diaphragm. Gentle movements ease out the stress and feel very nurturing. (If the person frequently suffers from anxiety, suggest that they apply warm sesame oil to their belly and then a hot pad or hot water bottle. Warm sesame oil to the feet before sleeping is also very helpful. If the person frequently experiences abdominal pain, suggest the same procedure using warm castor oil. This can help to soften scar tissue and dissolve old hard accumulations due to long-term constipation. If the pain is severe upon gentle touch, they should see a physician.)

Step Nine

Still at your friend's side, move to the waist level. Facing their torso, hold your hands about six inches above their belly, palms down.
Starting at the navel, make small clockwise circles over their body
with your hands, spiraling outward over their torso. Then bring the
left hand over the chest, up over the face and head, then the right hand
down over the hips, legs and feet, creating an imaginary capsule that
encircles your recipient roughly six inches from their body surface.
You can imagine this capsule being a protective shield filled on the
inside with healing light.

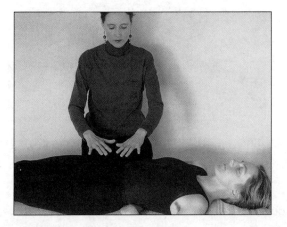

BENEFIT: Creating this type of protected space, the person feels safer
to experience the sensations and emotions that arise.

Step Ten

Standing behind the head of the your friend again, rest your thumbs on their third eye, a point midway between and slightly above the eyebrows. Rest your palms around both sides of the head.

Hold for a short time, breathing down into your belly.

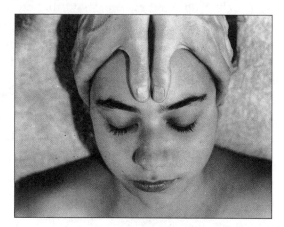

BENEFIT: This brings focus back to the face and head which is where the greater part of the massage takes place. It also helps you to be still and focus your own energy once again.

Although Steps One through Ten are preliminary to the main portion of the Ayurvedic Facial Massage Sequence, it is best if you have time to work through them thoroughly. If, however, you do not have time, at least spend a few minutes holding and focusing your attention on your friend's head, knees, ankles, forehead, then belly, keeping your focus and mentally creating a positive environment.

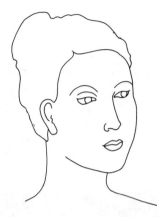

MASSAGE OF THE HEAD (*Shirobhyanga*)

When oil is applied to the head, it gets absorbed deep into the scalp through the roots of the hair. This nourishes, lubricates, and strengthens the hair roots and the skin of the scalp, preventing hair loss and premature greying. It improves circulation to the head, relaxing the muscles and nerve fibers. This helps to refresh both the mind and the body, relieving tension and fatigue and improving the complexion. This happens because massaging the head will increase fresh oxygen and glucose supply to the brain and improve the circulation of the spinal fluid around the brain and spinal cord. It also increases the release of hormones and enzymes necessary for the growth of the brain and relaxation of the body. Massage to the head increases the *prana,* the subtle aspect of the Vata dosha energy to the body.

Head massage is particularly beneficial before bathing in the morning, to gently awaken the nerves. In the evening it helps remove the stresses of the day and promotes peaceful sleep. Oiling the feet is also very helpful for deep, refreshing sleep as it tames Vata and banishes worries.

Step One

Point 1 is at the crown of the head on the midline. To find it easily and accurately, ask your friend to put their right hand over their forehead with the heel of the hand at the top of their nose with fingers pointing up over the head. Then, with their left hand, measure three finger widths back from the tip of the middle finger of their right hand. This is the crown point or *Mardhi* marma in the Ayurvedic tradition. This is the most therapeutic point on the head as it is where blood vessels, nerves, and lymphatics meet. Vata, Pitta, and Kapha doshas also meet here.

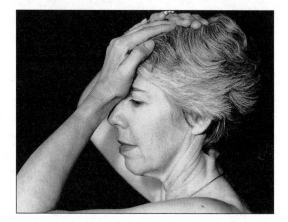

All marma points should be touched with great care, rubbing in gentle, small clockwise circles, gradually increasing, then gradually releasing pressure—spiraling in and spiraling out.

Apply warm oil from a squeeze bottle, then massage this marma point for 30-60 seconds, about the time it takes to do 35 clockwise circles. Remember this point and use it as a measuring reference for the other points.

BENEFITS:

(1) relieves neck tension and tension headaches

(2) facilitates the correction of deformities in the upper spine

(3) improves mental clarity and ability to concentrate
(4) pulls energy up in the body which can help give relief for hemorrhoids and pelvic congestion
(5) helps in the balancing and regulating of sensory and motor centers
in the brain

Step Two

Point 2 is three finger widths in front of the crown point, still on
the midline. (Remember to use the friend's hand as a reference, not
your own, or make appropriate allowances if you just "eyeball" it.)
This point is called *Brahma Randra* and is over the anterior fontanelle,
where babies have a soft spot. Sometimes you will feel a slight ridge
or depression where the bones come together. Rarely do the bones
not meet at this fontanelle point. However, if they do not, you may
just feel a leathery pad. Do not use pressure, only very gentle circular
movements.

Apply warm oil as before. Massage as in Step One—in small
clockwise circles, spiralling in then out for 30-60 seconds.

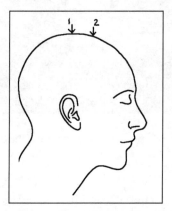

BENEFITS:

(1) regulates hormone release by stimulating the pituitary and pineal
glands

(2) facilitates the release of serotonin into the bloodstream which gives a sense of pleasure and satisfaction and elevates the mood

(3) increases the flow of cerebral-spinal fluid

(4) helps in the relief of insomnia

(5) helps to relieve frontal tension headaches

(6) strengthens the liver and digestive capacity to help normalize weight.

Step Three

Point 3 is four finger widths behind the crown point. It is called *Shiva Randra* and is over the posterior fontanelle. As with the anterior fontanelle mentioned in Step Two, you may feel a dip or ridge where the bones of the skull come together.

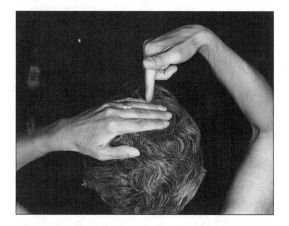

Massage as in Step One, again starting with the application of warm oil.

BENEFITS:

(1) facilitate the reduction of high blood pressure

(2) relieves dizziness and ringing in the ears

(3) creates alertness

(4) helps to improve the memory

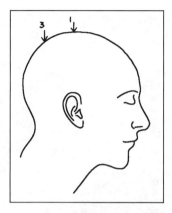

(5) helps to balance the activity of the pineal and pituitary glands
(6) helps relieve tension headaches and insomnia when used with points 1 and 2 and directs either side of the spine down to the mid-shoulder blade level

Step Four

Turn the friend's head to the left, cradling their head with your left hand. With the index and middle finger of your right hand find the bony bump behind the right ear lobe. This point is called *Karna* marma.

Massage this point in firm clockwise circular movements. Then, using your right hand, progress along the ridge of the skull toward the base of the neck, where the large neck muscles meet the skull. When you get to the base of the skull at the midline, switch hands to use your left hand to work up the back of the left side of the skull to the bump behind the left ear. Work from this point back to the right side, switching hands at the base of the skull midline. Repeat this back and forth process 2 more times. As you repeat this process, you will pass over two other marmas called *Manya* marmas. Give these special attention.

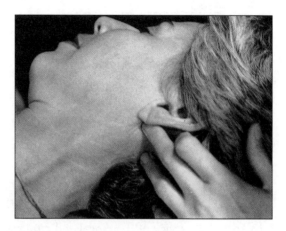

BENEFITS (from stimulating Karna marma):
(1) relaxes the muscles of the face and jaw
(2) relieves noises in the ears
(3) facilitates the clearing of middle ear congestion

BENEFITS (from stimulating Manya marma):
(1) relaxes the whole body via the spine reflexes
(2) relieves pain in the back of the head and neck tension
(3) can assist in improvement of hearing

Step Five

Keep the head turned to the left, cradling it in your left hand. Use all of the fingers of your right hand to stimulate the right side of the scalp in "zig zag" movements, from the back of the skull over the head to the hair line. Apply sufficient pressure so that skin is moved back and forth on the skull bones

Be sensitive to the individual. Thin people usually need less pressure and speed than heavier people with thick scalps to get the same result.

Work over the whole of the right side three times. Then turn the head to the right and repeat the process on the left side of the scalp. (Working with your left—or non-dominant—hand takes a little practice. However, it is very difficult to cross over and work with the right—or dominant—hand again on the left side.) Always support the

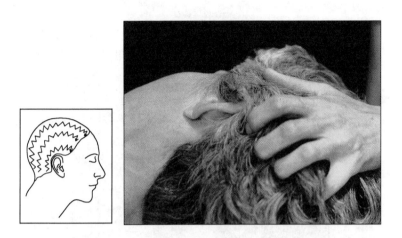

side of the head you are not working on so the recipient does not have to brace their neck to hold it in position for you.

Cradle the head with both hands so the neck is straight and the face up, to once again calm and ground the energy.

MASSAGE OF THE NECK AND UPPER CHEST

Step One

Raise the head slightly with your left hand and pinch down the spine from the base of the skull to the top of the shoulders using your right hand. Repeat twice.

At this point, moisten your fingertips with warm massage oil. Warm oil is more soothing and relaxing and penetrates the skin better. It also deepens the effect of the massage by nourishing the muscle tissue and lubricating the layers of connective tissue. Use sufficient oil from now on to allow your fingers to easily flow over the skin.

Step Two

Turn the head slightly to the left again, supporting it in your left hand. Find the bony point behind the earlobe again, but this time

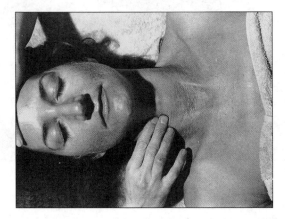

stroke down the large flat muscle that is attached to the skull at this point and wraps around the side of the neck and connects to the collar bone near the windpipe. This is the sterno-mastoid muscle. Repeat this stroking action one more time. Then turn the head slightly to the right and repeat the procedure on the left side.

Step Three

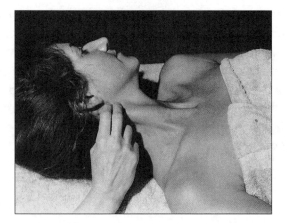

With the head back in the central position, tilt the chin slightly upward and stroke down either side of the windpipe from underneath the chin down to the collar bone. Repeat this step twice.

BENEFITS:

(1) loosens and tones the muscles on the front of the neck

(2) stimulates the thyroid gland which generates flow of fresh energy throughout the body

Step Four

Gently massage the mid point of the thyroid gland using very small clockwise circles.

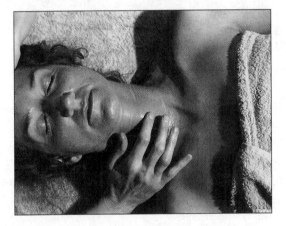

BENEFITS:

(1) helps in the regulation of the thyroid gland

(2) facilitates the verbalization of emotions

Step Five

Hook your thumb behind the notch at the top of the breast bone (sternum), in the natural hollow that is there. This point is called the *Jatru* marma. Press in under the bone and then gently release toward the windpipe, spiraling in and spiraling out. Do this twice. Sometimes this makes the recipient cough.

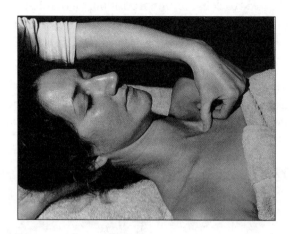

BENEFITS:

(1) clears chest congestion

(2) improves the tone of the voice

(3) facilitates the balance of the thyroid and parathyroid functions

(4) increases the circulation to the face

Then, gently tap down the breast bone using your finger tips to relieve tension and improve the opening of the rib cage during breathing. This stimulates the thymus gland which gives a boost to the immune system.

Step Six

With the second and third fingers of both your hands press the points where the collar bone meets the breast bone. These are the *Arshak* marmas. Press the point on one side, then the other.

BENEFITS: (from pressing the right Arshak marma)

(1) helps to improve liver and gall bladder function

(2) balances feelings of anger, pride, and frustration

(3) improves digestion generally

BENEFITS: (from pressing the left Arshak marma)

(1) improves spleen function

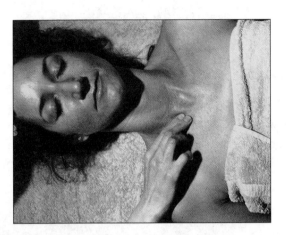

(2) helps to regulate blood sugar

(3) moderates mood swings

Using both hands together, stroke out from both these points along the top of the collar bone to the tips of the shoulders. Apply slight pressure to the tops of the shoulders, releasing quickly. Repeat once or twice.

Rest both of your hands on the tops of the shoulders. Relax. Focus on your breathing going deep into your belly. At this point, let your friend know that you are now going to start to work on their face. Most likely their eyes will be closed, so verbal ques prevent sparks of shock that can happen when you first touch this intimate part of the body.

When working directly on the face, use cold pressed, preservative free vegetable oil or combinations of oils. Top quality essential oils may be added for their aromatherapy effects (Check the list of suppliers listed at the back of this book). Be sure to dilute essential oils and do an allergy test on the arm as even the best quality ones can burn and cause long lasting irritation. Just because something is natural does not mean that it will never cause a problem. For an appropriate selection check in the chart that is included in the daily facial care section of this volume.

FACIAL MASSAGE

The smooth strokes release subtle tensions underneath the skin. Pressure points work on deeper tissues or reflexively on associated organ systems.

Step One

Cover your palms with a light amount of warm oil. Apply the oil using smooth strokes, starting from the midline of the chin and, using both of your entire hands, moving toward your temples.

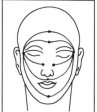 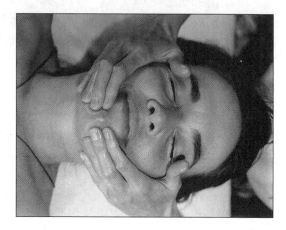

BENEFIT:
(1) Warm oil relaxes the muscles beneath the skin. It also "feeds" the skin. Sesame oil and essential oils are some of the few substances that actually penetrate the skin's outer layers.

Step Two

Place your fingers under the jaw, resting your thumbs on the jaw line. Ask your friend to open their mouth slightly. Manipulate the whole area under the chin and jaw by pressing up and releasing gently. Give special attention to the area at the root of the tongue and the tonsils, as a lot of tension collects there. This is particularly so if the

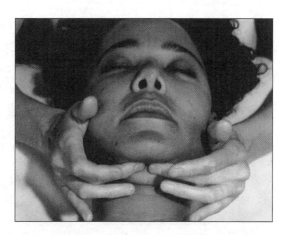

individual feels awkward about voicing their thoughts and feelings.

The musculature to the jaw holds a lot of tight habit patterns, some of which causes considerable discomfort in the neck as well as the face. The jaw muscle is actually the strongest muscle in the body. So tension here can trap a lot of body energy. If it is evident that there is a lot of jaw tension, ask the recipient to open their mouth as wide as possible while keeping the tip of their tongue behind their top front teeth. Encourage them to repeat this exercise 6 times a day. Reading aloud to oneself while holding a cork between the front teeth is another great technique to loosen the jaw. It is often used by actors who need mobility of expression.

BENEFITS:

(1) releases emotions

(2) releases jaw tension and the associated grinding of the teeth

(3) eases verbal communication

(4) massage of the temples helps to improve eyesight, creating a centered state of awareness and opens the mind to be receptive to new ideas

Step Three

Place your thumbs on the jaw at the chin with your index and third fingers underneath the jaw line. Apply pressure to the top and under-

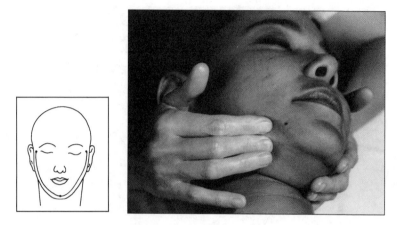

side of the jaw bone as you stroke up along the jaw line to the ears, then the temples. Lightly make small clockwise circles at the temples (clockwise meaning the direction a clock would move if placed face out on the person's skin. We use clockwise circles as they relieve tension better than other directions or types of pressure). Your fingers will be moving in opposite directions on either side of the head. This takes practice. Try one side at a time first.

The point at the temple is *Shankar* marma.

Repeat this stroke procedure twice more.

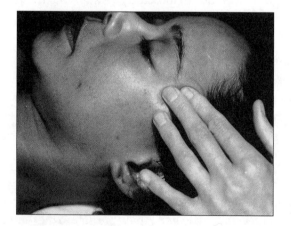

BENEFITS:

(1) relieves tension in the jaw

(2) relieves pressure around and in the eyeball

(3) assists in relieving tension headaches

(4) assists in reducing hyperactivity

(5) facilitates memory improvement

(6) opens the subconscious to suggestion or positive thought patterns

Step Four

Place your index fingers at the midpoint between the lower lip and the tip of the chin. Have your friend open their mouth slightly. Make small clockwise circles on this point.

Firmly stroke along the upper ridge of the jaw to just below the lower corners of the mouth. Make small clockwise circles again. Then continue to stroke along the jaw to the midpoint of the muscles that open and close the jaw. Make small circles again.

Stroke up the cheeks to the temples and massage as in Step Three. Repeat twice more.

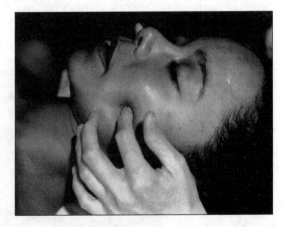

BENEFITS:

Point 1

(1) increases the circulation to the face

(2) relieves jaw tension

Point 2

(1) causes salivation, keeping the mouth moist (Massage can make you thirsty).

(2) softens wrinkles by improving muscle tone

Point 3

(1) relieves jaw tension, helping verbal expression and pain in the jaw, head, and neck (the TMJ syndrome)

Step Five

Place the tips of your index fingers midway between the nose and the middle of the upper lip. This point is called *Usta* marma. Press gently. Then stroke from this point out on both sides to the points just above the corners of the mouth, then under the cheek bones, to the top of the ear, over the ear, following the crease where the ear attaches to the head, to the bony bump behind the ear lobe. Repeat this procedure two more times. Pause at the points mentioned to apply slight pressure or small clockwise circular massage.

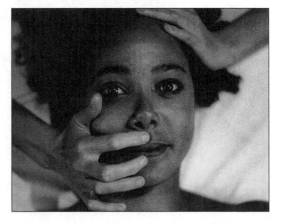

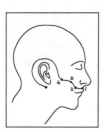

BENEFITS:

Point 1

(1) increases circulation to the brain

(2) improves alertness—is useful in relieving dizziness or nausea and reviving someone from fainting

(3) increases sexual desire

(4) softens horizontal lines that form after menopause or hysterectomy

Point 2

(1) moistens the mouth by causing salivation

(2) soothes wrinkles or helps their prevention by improving muscle tone at the corners of the mouth

Points 3 & 4

(1) opens the sinuses

(2) brings a rosy, healthy glow to the cheeks

(3) fills out the sunken tissues, softening the angles of the face

Step Six

Cover the left side of the top of the head with your left hand. Place your right index finger just above the flare of the right nostril. This point is called *Nasa* marma. Do small circular massage here, then stroke under the cheek bone, up to the temple, and over the ear as

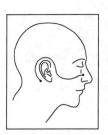

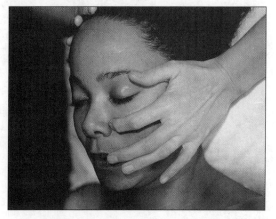

in Step Five. Repeat twice. Switch hands and repeat the same procedure on the left side.

BENEFITS:

Point 1

(1) improves the function of the opposite side of the brain.

(2) assists in the relief of asthma and bronchial congestion

Step Seven

Place the tips of the index fingers on either side of the nose midway between the corner of the eyes and the tip of the nostrils, on the nasal bones. This is the *Ganda* marma. Do small circular massage on the point on the right of the nose, then stroke over the cheek bone, pausing at the point directly below the midline of the eye (the pupil), making small clockwise circles, continuing on over the ear as before. End with a circular massage to the point behind the earlobe. Do this procedure on the left side. Then repeat, in alternation of both sides two more times.

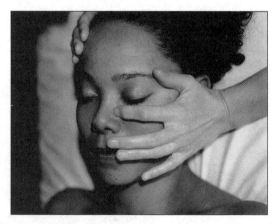

BENEFITS:

Point 1

(1) relieves sinus congestion and sinusitis

(2) brightens the eyes and relieves eye strain

(3) relieves congestion that causes bags to form under the eyes

(Steps Six and Seven can be worked on bilaterally, i.e. at the same time. But, one side at a time is more manageable as some of the points—especially for the sinuses—can be quite tender.)

Step Eight

Place your right index finger just below the inner corner of the right eye near to the nose. Rest your left hand over the left side of the head. Apply gentle pressure, then stroke along the lower bony surface that forms the eye socket, applying pressure at the points marked in the diagram. Do not pull on the skin, but glide, then press in tiny steps. End at the outer corner of the eye between the orbit and the eyeball. Press in gently at this point, called the *Apanga* marma. Repeat twice more, then three times on the opposite eye using the left hand.

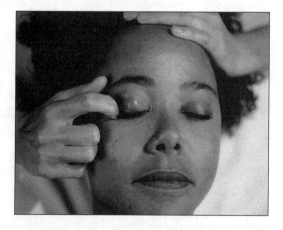

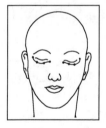

BENEFITS:

(1) makes the eyes water which releases emotions held in the eye sockets in a similar way to tears

(2) relieves tired eyes

(3) improves eyesight

(4) improves skin tone around the eye, relieving bags and darkness

Step Nine

Place the tips of both your index fingers at the tip of the nose. Stroke up the midline of the nose all the way to the top, then branch out either side to the point just below where the eyebrows begin on the upper bony surface that forms the eye socket. This point is *Kaninika* marma. Apply gentle pressure on both sides here, then continue along the upper ridge of the orbit emphasizing the points marked in the diagram, ending about ½ inch from the outer corner of the eye. Repeat twice more. You may want to do just one side at a time as this area can be sensitive, especially to clients with poor eyesight.

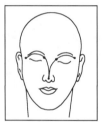
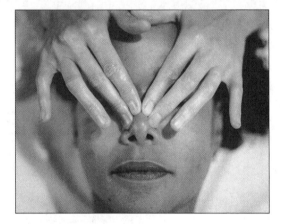

BENEFITS:

(1) releases energy to flow through the eye socket, the nose, and the center part of the face

(2) detoxifying effect on the liver

(3) helps in the release of repressed emotions, especially anger, frustration, grief

(4) relieves headaches due to eye strain

If the points covered in Steps Eight and Nine are very sensitive, *Netra Basti*, a process of bathing the eyes in warm ghee (clarified butter) is very helpful. This process is described in the section called "Special Ayurvedic Treatments." (pps. 237-42)

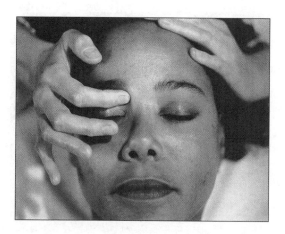

Step Ten
Starting at the inner (medial) end of the eyebrow, pinch along the eyebrow to its outer edge. Do this by keeping your index finger under the upper ridge of the eye sockets, using your thumb and index finger in a rolling action, index finger over the thumb, then thumb over the index finger. Repeat once more.

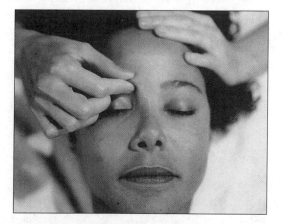

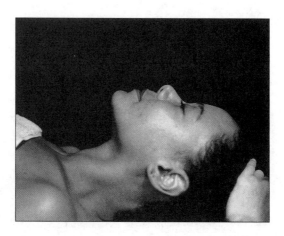

BENEFITS:
(1) releases tension held throughout the body, especially in the upper ridge of the eye socket
(2) stimulates the delicate muscles around the temples to help release crow's feet
(3) helps the eyes
(4) helps to nourish and relax the nervous system

Step Eleven

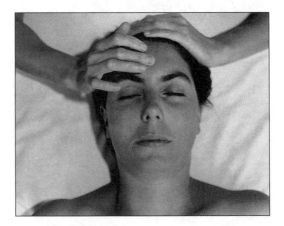

Stroke from the tip of the nose to the area of the third eye, which is slightly above the midpoint between the eyebrows. This point is *Ajna* marma. Massage this area in gentle, clockwise motions for 60-90 seconds.

BENEFITS:
(1) relieves headaches over the eyes
(2) assists to relieve emotional tension
(3) balances the subtle energies of the body
(4) clears perceptions
(5) brings peace to the mind

Sometimes people feel very strong energy at this point. Ask if your friend feels this. If they do, ask them to direct this feeling towards the center of the body and from there let it expand, energizing every muscle and organ system to help them stay grounded.

Application of the cream from milk to the forehead creates pleasurable feelings. Moist clay packs here help to cool the whole system. A drop of essential oil of sandalwood applied to *Ajna* marma (third eye area) helps the mind be clear and peaceful, better prepared for meditation.

Step Twelve

With the fingers of one hand shaped in a claw-like position and the opposite hand supporting the head, make zig-zag motions from one side of the forehead to the other. As you zig-zag from left to right support the left side of the head, and vice versa. Supporting the head prevents the sides of the neck from bracing.

Zig-zag twice more, then stroke twice across the forehead again, this time using the heel of the hand. Zig-zag twice, then stroke once from left to right, then right to left.

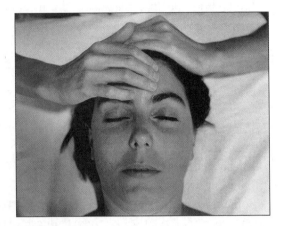

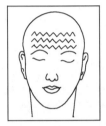

BENEFITS:
(1) brings warmth and relaxation to the muscles of the forehead
(2) builds muscle tone helping to prevent lines and wrinkles
(3) helps improve eyesight
(4) increases the power of concentration

Step Thirteen

Repeat the same stroking procedure as in Step Eleven, from the tip of the nose, up along the sides of the nose to the forehead and continue up the midline of the forehead to the hair line. Massage in small circular motions out to the right and left along the hairline, over the ears to the back of the head. Let your fingers meet at the base of the skull.

Now massage up the back of the head, either side of the midline, with the same circular movements upwards and outwards. Continue over the top of the head to the front hair line. Repeat, this time starting from the hair line.

Tensions are often held at the hairline as it is the boundary between the face which is visible to others and the scalp, which is not. On the midline of the skull there are energy centers like the chakras, or energy wheels, that are found on the main trunk of the body. Massage over these points stimulates deep centers of the brain and helps to balance the body physically, mentally, and emotionally.

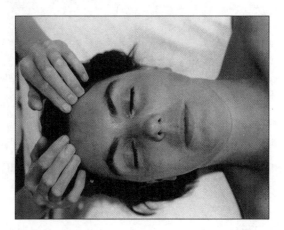

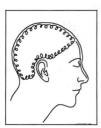

BENEFITS:
(1) opens a flow of energy down into the face
(2) relaxes and invigorates the muscles of the forehead
(3) relieves head pain
(4) stimulates chakras in the head

EAR MASSAGE

Cradle the head so that it is slightly turned to the left and supported by the left hand. Maintain this position for the 5 steps of the ear massage.

Step One

Hold the right earlobe between the thumb and index finger. With a rolling, gentle squeezing motion, move along the outer edge of the ear to the point where the ear connects to the head. Repeat this twice.

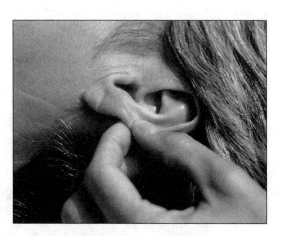

BENEFITS:
(1) relieves tension and can assist in correcting deformities of the spine
(2) stimulates the central nervous system

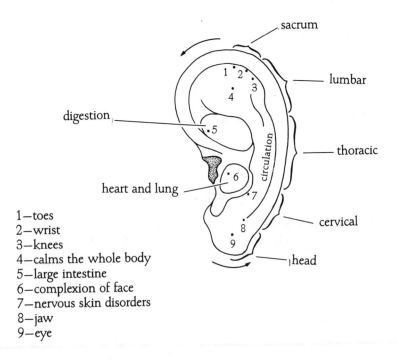

1—toes
2—wrist
3—knees
4—calms the whole body
5—large intestine
6—complexion of face
7—nervous skin disorders
8—jaw
9—eye

Step Two
Work in a similar fashion along the middle ridge of the ear. Repeat twice.

BENEFIT:
(1) facilitates improvement in circulation

Step Three
Use the tips of your index fingers to rub the inner most part of the ear and the ear hole. Applying oil around the ear hole can help to alleviate ringing in the ears. Pouring warm sesame oil to fill the ear is a deeper form of treatment for this disorder. (This should not be done if infection is present.)

Step Four
Rub the ear where it attaches to the head, starting behind the lobe and working your way up behind the ear to the point where the top portion of the pinna attaches to the head. Check the ear massage diagram for direction.

BENEFITS:
(1) helps to balance the Vata dosha by having an indirect effect on the colon
(2) works on the energy to the small and large intestine
(3) stimulates the brain
(4) lowers high blood pressure
(5) if pressed hard, creates a natural "high"

Step Five
Strongly flick the ear to and fro using all the fingers shaped into a loose paddle 10 times. (If this process seems too vigorous for your friend, rub the ear with your whole hand until it is warm.)

BENEFITS:
(1) strongly energizes the kidneys which helps with low back pain and improves stamina

(2) improves circulation and has a warming effect on the body

(3) helps excretory functions which is helpful in removing toxins released by the massage process

Turn the head now to the right, supporting the head with your right hand. Repeat all steps for the left ear.

Briefly lay the palms of your hands over each ear, holding in the warmth and energy that has been produced in this process.

CLOSING MASSAGE

Rub your hands together until they are really warm. Place them over your friend's eyes. Heat energy from your hand can first be felt entering the eyes and deep into the skull, then gradually penetrating into the body. Direct your friend's attention to this. Ask if they feel the warmth. Then ask them to direct this experience throughout the body.

Finally, rest your thumbs over the closed eyelids, your palms over their forehead, and the tips of your middle fingers closing their ears. This encloses them in a quiet dark space for a few minutes to be with their inner experience before they once again face the world.

Gently release your hands, touch both shoulders and let your friend know that the massage is complete. Tell them to take their time,

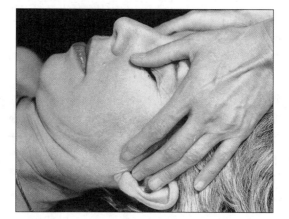

and encourage them to move slowly when they feel ready. Take a few minutes to share experiences together. Remind them to try and be in a calm, relaxed environment for the next hour, or at least to avoid confrontations, crowds, noise, or heavy traffic.

Testimonials for Facial Massage

"The idea of Ayurvedic facials appealed to me because I was hopeful that eastern healing techniques could relax my head and neck where I hold a lot of tension.

The experience of the Ayurvedic facial, however, far surpassed my expectations. Muscles released throughout my body, not just in my face. The relief of feeling painful knots dissolve in my head, neck, and shoulders was exquisite. Unconscious patterns of holding let go, smoothing all lines and furrows.

I left with a softer, younger, happier face, and a looser body. The memory of relaxation is something I strive to recreate everyday, teaching my muscles to release their grip.

The Ayurvedic facial is the high light of my week."

Michelle Herman

"Melanie Sachs' work was wonderful. Something magical happened as my body let go and it's energy shifted me into a roomier and more peaceful place in my body."

Deb Bergeron

SPECIAL AYURVEDIC TREATMENTS

Traditionally used for their healing qualities, these special Ayurvedic techniques have the additional benefit of enhancing the appearance. Working deeply on the central nervous system, they activate the centers of the brain, having both a relaxing and rejuvenating effect on the entire body. The result is what I call "discovering the original face," a face (and mind state) that is soft, open, gentle, vital, and centered. Such techniques invoke beauty from the deepest levels of our being.

Both preventive and therapeutic in effect, the techniques that follow can raise to a conscious level deep seated memories, fears, and anxieties that keep tensions locked into the body. At the same time, they are so wonderfully gentle that they can help to clear away the somatic aspect of life's traumas, thus being truely transformative without risk of creating heightened vulnerability and re-traumatization. At the same time, care should be given to provide a protected, loving environment before, during, and after treatment.

NETRA BASTI

Netra Basti means washing the eye with medicated oils. It is an ancient treatment from India to relieve the tensions that are trapped in the eye socket that can result in poor eyesight, pain, fatigue, and that sunken, sallow look. Traditionally, this treatment is used to improve eyesight and nourish the nervous system via the eyeball as it connects directly to the brain. We have found it also brings an incredibly rich lustre to the eyes, soothes away wrinkles, enhances color and depth perception, creates a sense of ease and acceptance, and promotes a deep feeling of contentment.

This treatment is deep acting and the emotional results are unpredictable, so it is important that it be done in a calm, quiet, protected environment with care and support. Do not leave the recipient alone at any point during the treatment. Afterwards encourage your friend/ recipient to give themselves a minimum of two hours quiet time away from the stresses of bright lights, loud noise, crowds, or emotional confrontations. This process opens your field of vision allowing impressions to flow deep into your visual memory banks. Let those impressions be pleasant ones.

To give Netra Basti, you need:

(1) ½ cup of ghee or clarified butter (see recipe) in ceramic or glass container

(2) 1 cup of whole wheat flour mixed with approximately 1/2 cup of water to make two dough balls of earlobe consistency

(3) 2 small bowls, one to hold the dough, the other to catch the ghee after application

(4) a tablespoon

(5) facial tissue

(6) small bowl of hot water or a small sized crock pot to keep the ghee warm

Set up your equipment on a small tray for ease of access. The temperature of the ghee should be such that if you swish your finger in it, it should feel just warm. Temperature of oily substances is best measured by this swishing. Just placing your finger in the ghee will give you a false impression of its actual temperature.

Check that the recipient has removed contact lenses if they wear them. Explain the procedure. Ask them to lie down on their back. Make them warm and comfortable so they can relax more easily. A pillow under the knees helps relieve strain some people may feel in their lower backs. A hot pack on the belly or feet feels extra special on cold types.

Step One

Start with a brief polarity balancing as described in the massage section, holding first the head, shoulders, knees, ankles, and then the head and belly together.

Step Two

Proceed by giving a brief stroking massage to the face using only enough oil to allow your fingers to move freely. Follow the outward and upward strokes as shown in the diagrams in the facial massage section. Wipe off any excess oil around the eyes, as this will interfere with the seal of the dough ring that will be pressed around the eye socket.

Step Three

Form half the dough into a small doughnut-shaped ring that will fit around the eye socket.

Begin with the right eye. Turn the recipient's head slightly to the left so the eye is looking directly upward. Support their head on the left side with a rolled-up towel. Place the doughnut around the eye socket, pressing it firmly toward the skin on the inside and outside of the ring.

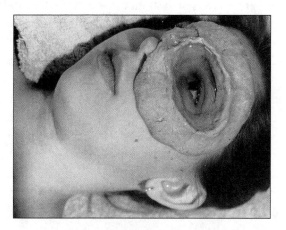

Step Four

Pour ½ teaspoon of ghee (that feels just barely warm to your finger) in the outer corner of the eye. Ask if the temperature is comfortable. (This is a relative perception which varies from person to person, so it is always best to ask. If it seems too warm as reported by them, allow the ghee to cool by pouring it back and forth in two containers. If not hot enough, it takes only a brief moment for ghee to get hot again. Again, always check with the finger swishing method first.) If the temperature is richly warm and comfortable, spoon in another 4-5 tablespoons of the ghee so the eye and eye lashes are completely covered. Some people like the other eye covered to block out light and other visual distraction. Use either your fingers or folded wash cloth to gently hold the eye closed.

Step Five

The person may keep the eye closed or open it. The ghee may sting or burn a little at first. This should pass if the eye tears as they blink several times. Once they are comfortable with the eye open, the eye can be gently moved in the eight directions of the compass and rolled clockwise and counter-clockwise. These movements should be slow and gentle so as not to strain the muscles. Close and rest the eye as needed. Sometimes the opposite eye will tear, so have a tissue handy.

Occasionally this experience brings up suppressed traumatic memories or feelings. Be supportive and willing to stop the treatment if necessary. Holding the top of your friend's head with your palms is often comforting or even just touching the top of the head. Usually the same emotions do not come up with each eye so you can encourage them to try the other eye. Sometimes this will calm down the situation. Keep the ghee in for 20 minutes. This is rather a strange and slightly involved procedure and can, in itself, be anxiety provoking. Explain the process step by step and be prepared to work slowly.

Step Six
Remove the ghee by making a small indentation on the lateral edge of the doughnut ring so that it acts like a spout. Turn your friend's head slowly toward you to pour the ghee out into one of the small bowls.

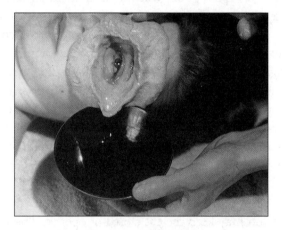

Remove the dough and wipe the excess ghee off with a tissue.

Repeat Steps One through Six for the left eye.

Sometimes people of Pitta constitution or people with a lot of excess Pitta in their system have the whites of their eyes turn a little red. If this persists, apply a few drops of pure rose water or cucumber juice to the eye. Check eye care section, p. 142 for other suggestions.

BENEFITS reported from doing Netra Basti:

(1) improved memory

(2) increased ease in speaking a foreign language

(3) remembering visual traumas in a way that is gentle and supported through the process

(4) greater ease in seeing

(5) release of tension throughout the body

(6) softness in appearance

Making Ghee or Clarified Butter

Put one pound of unsalted butter into a saucepan. Heat slowly until the butter is completely melted and starts to boil. Reduce heat and simmer.

At first the melted butter is cloudy and a white fatty scum rises to the top. The sound of the butter boiling is like the low hiss of water. The scum will then fall to the bottom as the melted butter starts to clear and a sediment is more visible at the bottom. Continue to simmer until the sediment becomes golden brown and the rest of the liquid becomes golden in color and clear. The sound you will hear will go from a hissing to the sound of crackling, like deep frying oil. Good ghee smells like popcorn. Turn off the heat and allow it to cool for 10 minutes.

Place a strainer lined with cheesecloth or muslin over an earthenware or glass jar. Pour the ghee through the strainer, making an effort not to allow any of the sediment to leave the saucepan. As the ghee cools it will solidify or become semi-aqueous. Refrigeration is not necessary.

Testimonial for Netra Basti

"Although I was drawn to this treatment when I read about it, the closer the time came for the treatment the more worried about it I became. Hot butter in my eyes?! Really now!

But as soon as Melanie began the treatment, all my anxieties were relieved.

All I felt was a warm, gentle caressing of my eyelids and when I opened my eyes to the butter, the warmth continued feeling wonderful. Afterwards my eyes were very relaxed. I felt I could actually see better—with less strain.

I feel that, as a result of the treatment, I was able to get some insight into my visual problems so that I could start making some changes on the emotional level."

Margaret Thompson

NASYA

Nasya is a nasal administration of medicated powders or liquid drops. The powders or drops can be of a calming nature that helps to promote sleep or relaxation, or more cleansing and stimulating in nature, or purely nutritive. Here we use liquid drops that are more cleansing in action. By cleansing we mean cleansing the sinus cavities but also clearing the area of the head and neck of excess Vata energy—that which causes pain and tension. Vata energy in the head is known as *"prana."* Prana energy relates to higher cerebral, sensory, and motor functions and movement in the kidneys.

Classically, this type of treatment is used for clearing the sinuses, reducing pain in the face, head, and neck, and helping kidney function. From the beauty point of view it definitely reduces dark rings under the eyes, a pinched look in the sinuses, and/or a sunken or puffy look around the eyes. It is a simple technique, but its effects run deep, both physically and emotionally. Please always observe these contraindications:

Never do Nasya . . .
   (1) after a hot bath
   (2) after eating a meal
   (3) after having sexual intercourse

(4) after drinking alcohol

(5) during menstruation or pregnancy

The equipment you will need to do Nasya is . . .

(1) quarter of a cup of sesame oil

(2) glass eye dropper with a rubber end

(3) fine grater or blender

(4) 3″ long piece of good, fresh ginger root

(5) a small amount of clean water

(6) facial tissues

(7) hot water bottle or hot water and a wash cloth if a bottle is
not available

There are three main types of nasya that are classified according
to their action: 1) *Shodhan,* or cleansing Nasya, 2) *Shamana,* or paci-
fying Nasya, and 3) *Bruhan,* or nourishing nasya. Shodhan, or cleansing Nasya, has the most dramatic effect on the appearance, so I have
selected one form of Shodhan to describe the Nasya process in detail.

PREPARATION of the GINGER CLEANSING NASYA (or *SHODHAN*) SOLUTION

Step One

Grate the ginger using a fine grater or blender. Squeeze out the juice
from the pulp into a small bowl. (If you have a juicer, this will also
work.) Strain the juice through a fine meshed strainer.

Step Two

Add a pinch of brown sugar and a dash of water per 2 tablespoons
of ginger juice. The sugar stops the ginger from burning. (This solution should be stored in the refrigerator when not being used.)

Step Three

Wrap the hot water bottle in a towel to keep it warm. Or, prepare
the hot water with a wash cloth so that it is ready for use.

Step Four

Warm the sesame oil

Step Five

Arrange all of the equipment to be within easy reach. Make sure the room is quiet and warm.

The NASYA PROCEDURE:

Step One

Have your friend lie on their back and perform the Preliminary massage as per instructions in facial massage section.

Step Two

Give a vigorous facial massage with warm sesame oil. Clockwise circular motions will relieve stress in the facial tissue. However, the main purpose of the massage, at this point, is simply to increase circulation and work the oil into the skin.

Step Three

Place a facial tissue on both sides of the face so that the nose is the only exposed area. Lay the hot water bottle or hot pack (wash cloth) on one side of the face for a short period of time and then repeat on the other side. Keep applying heat in this way until the face is really rosy and the oil has gone into the skin.

Step Four

Place a rolled up towel under the neck so that their head is supported and slightly cocked back, their nostrils pointing upwards.

Step Five

Apply 3 to 5 drops of the ginger juice solution into the right nostril with the eye dropper. Massage the sinus areas above and below the right eye. The eye may tear, indicating some emotional release. They may also feel energy dancing over their face. Use smooth massage strokes to ground this energy. Ask when they are ready for application to the left nostril. Proceed in the same manner as you did on

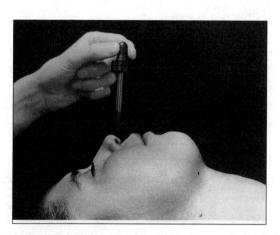

the right side. Rest briefly after procedure.

You can give this treatment once a week over a four week period, increasing the amount by two drops per week. For example: week 1, 4 drops; week 2, 6 drops; and so on up to a maximum of 10 drops per nostril.

Step Six

Take your time. When the process is complete, support your friend's shoulders as they sit up. Support the sternum with one hand and use your other hand to stroke down their spine. Have them move slowly and suggest that they take their time with things over the next hour.

Nasya can be done like this 3 days in a row or every 3-4 days on an ongoing basis.

BENEFITS: (reported)
(1) feeling relaxed and recharged all over
(2) relief of tension patterns around the chest
(3) better and longer sleep
(4) relief of chronic neck pain
(5) feel alert and have more energy

(6) look younger

(7) have less stress held in the face

Regarding the use of *Shamana* nasya, this is useful to calm the nervous system and still the mind for restful sleep. Use vacha or siddha soma oil.

To do *Bruhan* Nasya requires special herbal oils designed to improve all of the senses.

Testimonial for Nasya

"During the treatment I felt a tremendous sense of emotional release which was facilitated by my body's reaction to the ginger, as well as the gentleness of the therapist.

My sleep that night was the best in a long time and the next day the dark rings under my eyes, a chronic condition, had completely disappeared."

Carol Hoy

SHIRO DHARA

Shiro Dhara is the process of running a fine stream of warm sesame oil on the "third eye" area of the forehead for a period of approximately half an hour. Classically, it was used for cases of pain and stress, particularly but not exclusively, in the face, head, neck, and shoulders. Stimulation to the "third eye" area affects deep centers in the brain that release brain chemicals; one of which is serotonin, a chemical that gives us the feeling of pleasure and relaxation. It also frees the subtle energies of channels situated along the spine that help to calm and clear the mind.

The equipment you will need is:

    (1) massage table

    (2) blanket and pillow

    (3) traditional shiro dhara pot or separatory funnel with ring and stand (available through chemical and chemistry equipment suppliers)

(4) large bowl
(5) one-quart of warm cold-pressed sesame oil

The person lies on their back on the massage table under a blanket to keep them warm. Some people with back problems will feel more comfortable with a pillow under their knees.

Step One

Give the Preliminary Massage as described in the facial massage section. Then apply warm oil to the face in deliberate strokes and in accordance with Step One in the Facial Massage section. (This type of energy balancing work is traditionally given in Ayurveda before any kind of a more specific procedure.)

Step Two

Have the client scoot back on the table so that their head is slightly over the edge of the table. A rolled towel under the neck will provide a more comfortable tilt to the head.

Step Three

Arrange the bowl on the floor to catch the oil.

Step Four

Warm the oil and pour the first portion of it into the separatory funnel.

Step Five

Position the funnel on a table, or stand so that the tip of the funnel will allow the oil to drip on the "third eye" area in the middle of the forehead. Check to make sure the oil is not too warm for the client.

Step Six

Release the valve on the funnel so that a continuous fine stream of oil plays on the "third eye", then flows over the forehead through the hair along the midline of the head and then falls into the bowl.

There are energy centers on the top of the head that correspond to the seven energy wheels or chakras on the midline of the body.

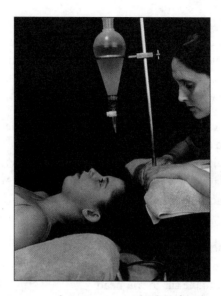

Warm oil flowing over these areas on the head, calms and balances the energies in the body that cause pain and stress.

Step Seven

Stay with the client at all times and keep checking that the oil is flowing in the right place. Refill the funnel with the rest of the oil when the funnel is about half empty. In India, this procedure is sometimes done for longer periods, in which case the oil is re-warmed and used again.

Step Eight

When the funnel is empty, wipe off the excess oil from the client's forehead and hair and tell them to move slowly when they are ready.

It is also useful to suggest to them that for several hours they try to remain in fairly calm surroundings and to avoid stressful encounters where possible.

BENEFITS (as seen and reported):

    (1) Opening and soothing to the face and forehead

(2) trapped energy released throughout the body

(3) strong flow of psychic impressions and lucid dreaming

(4) clearing of the mind so decisions can be made more easily and more information handled with ease

Testimonial for Shiro Dhara

"Shiro Dhara is very calming and relaxing for my body during the treatment. Afterwards my mind is very clear and all the extraneous internal chatter is gone."

Karuna Fluhart

KARNA PURANA

This is filling the ears with warm sesame oil. It is most easily done with the help of a partner, but once the amount of oil needed to fill a particular ear has been measured, it is possible to do this process yourself.

The equipment you will need is:

1) small pot

2) hot plate or heat source

3) spoon

4) towels

Procedure:

1) Have your friend lie on their side with a rolled-up towel to support the head. For the right ear, have the left arm straight behind your friend's torso, the right arm bent and in front, supporting the chest and shoulders. Have the left leg straight and the right leg bent with the knee on the ground/mattress to support the pelvis and hips. Use pillows under the bent knee or make adjustments to the pose if necessary. The aim here is for the body to be as comfortable and relaxed as possible. Whatever works towards that end, do.

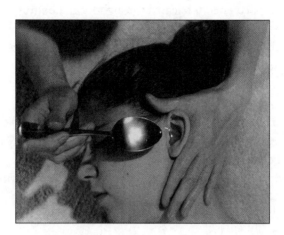

2) Take warm sesame oil and fill the right ear as full as possible without spilling.

3) Using your index finger, massage behind the ear, from top to bottom, finishing behind the ear lobe.

4) Allow the oil to remain in the ear for a minimum of 10 minutes and a maximum of 20 minutes.

5) Empty the oil out of the ear into a bowl having your friend turn the head and slowly roll onto the back. Wipe any excess oil from the ear.

6) Repeat on the opposite side.

BENEFITS of Karna Purana include:

      1) relieves itching and dryness in the ears

      2) reduces Vata dosha to clear the sense of hearing

      3) useful in relieving ringing in the ears

A FINAL NOTE

The power of *Ayurvedic Beauty Care* comes from the ability to become familiar with our basic nature. The secret is to accept our own uniqueness and be willing to fully respond to our needs in a truly nurturing fashion. When such action is both loving and intelligent it will naturally evoke from within the beautiful manifestation of creation that is completely who we are. Such an approach—one of understanding and kindness—to ourselves, is the seed of the only kind of beauty that has any lasting value: inner beauty.

Inner Beauty only shines brighter with time; its essence being to benefit everyone.

ABOUT THE AUTHOR

Melanie Sachs is internationally known for her ongoing work in promoting sound preventative health care and beauty practices. Conventionally trained as an Occupational Therapist and having learned from some of the finest teachers of oriental healing in both Britain and America, especially in the areas of Macrobiotics and Ayurveda, she is certified as an Ayurvedic Lifestyle Management counselor.

With her husband, Bob, Melanie is co-director of Diamond Way Health Associates. They and their children, Kai Ling, Christina, and Jabeth live in Albuquerque, New Mexico.

RESOURCE BIBLIOGRAPHY

Aromatherapy:

Keller, Eric. *Aromatherapy Handbook.* (Healing Arts Press, Rochester, Vermont, 1991)

Price, Shirley. *Aromatherapy for Common Ailments.* (Fireside, Simon and Schuster, Inc, New York, 1991)

Tisserand, Maggie. *Aromatherapy For Women.* (Wellingborough, Northamptonshire, NN8 2RQ, England, Thorsons Publishers Limited, 1985)

Tisserand, Robert, *Aromatherapy: To Heal and Tend the Body.* (Lotus Press, Twin Lakes, Wisconsin, 1988)

Tisserand, Robert. *The Art of Aromatherapy.*(Saffron Walden, Essex, CB10 1JP, England, C.W. Daniel Company Ltd., 1989)

Ayurveda and Ayurvedic Massage:

Bhagwandash, Vaidya. *Massage Therapy in Ayurveda.* (Concept Publishing Company, New Delhi, 1934)

Chopra, Dr. Deepak. *Perfect Health.* (Harmony Books, New York, 1991)

Frawley, Dr. David. *Ayurvedic Healing.* (Passage Press, Morson Publishing, Salt Lake City, Utah, 1989)

Johari, Harish. *Ancient Ayurvedic Massage.* (Munshiram Manoharlal Publishers, Ltd., New Delhi, India, 1984)

Lad, Dr. Vasant. *Ayurveda: The Science of Self-Healing.* (Lotus Press, Twin Lakes, Wisconsin, 1984)

Lad, Dr. Vasant and Frawley, Dr. David. *Yoga of Herbs.* (Lotus Press, Twin Lakes, Wisconsin, 1986)

Pathah. *Pandit Ram Raksha. Therapeutic Guide to Ayurvedic Medicine.* (Shree Baidyanath Ayurved Bhawan Private, Ltd., India)

Svoboda, Robert E. *Ayurveda: Life, Health, and Longevity.* (Arkana, The Penguin Group, Harmondsworth, Mddx., ENGLAND, 1992)

Svoboda, Robert E. *Prakruti: Your Ayurvedic Constitution.* (160 Washington Ave. SE, Albuquerque, New Mexico 87108, Geocom Limited, 1988). Distributed by Lotus Press, Twin Lakes, Wisconsin

Thakkur, Chandrashekhar G.. *Introduction to Ayurveda.* (Times of India Press, Bombay, India, 1965)

Diet:

Ballentine, Dr. Rudolph. *Diet and Nutrition; a holistic approach.* (Himalayan International Institute, Honesdale, PA, 1978)

Colbin, Annamarie. *Food and Healing.* (Ballantine Books, div. of Random House, New York, 1986)

Dunne, Lavon J. *Nutrition Almanac.* (McGraw Hill Publishing, 1990)

Morningstar, Amadea. *The Ayurvedic Cookbook.* (Lotus Press, Twin Lakes, Wisconsin, 1990)

Tiwari, Maya, and Esko, Wendy, and Kushi, Aveline. *Diet for Natural Beauty.* (Japan Publishing, New York and Tokyo, 1991)

Beauty (general):

Buchman, Dian Dincin. *Feed Your Face.* (The Old Piano Factory, 43 Gloucester Crescent, London NW1, Gerald Duckworth & Co. Ltd., 1973)

Hampton, Aubrey. *Natural Organic Hair and Skin Care.* (4419 N. Manhattan, Ave., Tampa, Fl. 33614, Organica Press, 1987)

Kenton, Leslie. *The Joy of Beauty.* (Arrow Books, Ltd., London, 1989)

Wagner, Lindsay and Klein, Robert M. *Lindsay Wagner's New Beauty: The Acupressure Facelift.* (Prentice Hall Press, New York, London, Toronto, Sydney, Tokyo, 1987)

Exercise and Relaxation:

Chia, Mantak and Maneewan. *Awaken Healing Light of the Tao.* (Healing Tao Books, Huntington, N.Y., 1993)

de Langre, Jacques. *The First Book of DO-IN.* (Happiness press, Magalia, CA., 1971)

de Langre, Jacques. *The Second Book of Do-IN 2.* (Happiness Press, Magalia, CA 1974)

Hashimoto, Keizo. *Sotai Natural Exercise.* (available through Vega Institute, Oroville, CA)

Kushi, Michio. *The Book of Do-In: Exercise for Physical and Spiritual Development.* (Tokyo, Japan, Japan Publications, Inc., 1979)

Oki, Masahiro. *Oki Yoga for Easy Childbirth and Feminine Health Care.* (East West Centre, Amsterdam, Holland, 1978)

Pinckney, Callan. *Callanetics.* (Avon Books, New York, 1984)

Reed Gach, Michael and Marco, Carolyn. *Acu-Yoga.* (Japan Publications, Inc., Tokyo and New York, 1981)

Stone, Justin. *Tai Chi Chih.* (Satori Resources, San Leandro, CA, 1984)

Sutton, Dr. Marcea. *In Harmony: Resolving Stress.* Zivah Publishers, Albuquerque, New Mexico, 1991.

Trager, Dr. Milton. *Trager Mentastics: Movement as a Way to Agelessness.* (Station Hill Press, Barrytown, N.Y.)

Tulku, Tarthang. *Kum Nye Relaxation, Part 1: Theory, Preparation, Massage.* (2425 Hillside Ave., Berkley, California, Dharma Publishing, 1978)

Herbs and Oils:

Garland, Sarah. *The Herb & Spice Book.* (Mortimer House, 37-41 Mortimer House, London W1N 7RJ, Francis Lincoln Publishers, Ltd., 1979)

Frawley, Dr. David and Lad, Dr. Vasant. *Yoga of Herbs.* (Lotus Press, Twin Lakes, Wisconsin, 1986)

Lawless, Julia. *Encyclopedia of Essential Oils.* (Element Books, Ltd., Shaftesbury, Dorset, England, 1992)

Rose, Jeanne. *Jeanne Rose's Herbal Body Book.* (Perigee Books, Putnam Publishing Group, New York, 1976)

Tierra, Michael. *Planetary Herbology.* (Lotus Press, Twin Lakes, Wisconsin, 1988)

Wood, Magda Ironside, editor. *"All You Need To Know About HERBS."* (58 Old Compton Street, London, W1V 5PA, Marshall Cavendish Ltd., 1973)

Light, Sound, Color, and Gems:

Anderson, Mary. *Chromatherapy and How It Works.* (Aquarian Press, ENGLAND)

Chogyam, Ngakpa. *Rainbow of Liberated Energy.* (Element Books Ltd., Shaftesbury, Dorset, ENGLAND)

Gimbel, Theo. *Form, Sound, Colour and Healing.* (C.W. Daniel Company, Ltd., Saffron Walden, England, 1987)

Raphaell, Katrina. *Crystal Healing.* (Aurora Press, Santa Fe, N.M., 1987)

Meditation:

Trungpa, Chogyam. *Shambhala: The Sacred Path of the Warrior.* (Shambhala Publications, Inc., Boulder, CO. 1984)

GLOSSARY

agni—the cosmic force of transformation. Also, the power of digestion for food, emotions, and sensations.

ama—internal toxins that are usually the result of incomplete digestion or elimination of foods or emotions, or improper metabolic function.

apatarpana—well toned and clean.

asthi—bone tissue.

atapa—sun or moon bathing.

aura—the body's subtle energy field which is produced and sustained by ojas.

basma—a medicine made by oxidizing metals or minerals to form their ash.

baspa sweda—steam bath using a steam box.

dhana sweda—hot shower of water along the spine.

dhatu—literally means "that which supports life;" one of the seven basic body tissues that nourish each other.

dosha—literally means "fault" or "mistake." A dosha is one of the three subtle forces that hold the five elements together in living things and supports their functioning. They are known as Vata (combining ether and air), Pitta (combining fire and water), and Kapha (combining earth and water).

drava sweda—hot herbal bath.

essential oil—the essence or life blood of a plant that carries its fragrance and holds its healing power.

ghee—clarified butter, highly valued in Ayurveda for its medicinal uses both internally and externally.

guna—quality or attribute of a given substance or phenomena.

hara—the Japanese term for the energetic center of the physical body according to oriental medicine.

hastavagaha—hot herbal hand bath.

kapha—earth-water constitution, the force in the body responsible for stability and lubrication.

karna purana—oleation of the ear canal.

kichadi—an easily digested stew of rice, split hulled mung beans, spices, and vegetables.

kshud—fasting from food or taking a mono-diet (such as one type of grain, a juice, even kichadi).

majja—bone marrow, nerve tissue—that which fills bony spaces.

malas—waste products of the body, such as urine, feces, perspiration.

mamsa—muscle tissue.

marma—energy pressure point.

marut—taking fresh air.

meda—adipose tissue, fat.

nasya—nasal application of medicated oils, herbal powders, or milk.

netra basti—bathing the eye with ghee or medicated oil.

ojas—the essential vitality of the body. It supports the aura, connects the energy of the mind to the body and supports immunity.

padavagaha—foot massage.

pancha karma—literally means "five cleansing actions." These cleansing actions include vamana (therapeutic vomiting), basti (nutritive, cleansing, or rejuvenating enemas), nasya (nasal applications), virechana (therapeutic purgation), and rakta moksha (blood purification).

Pitta—fire and water constitution, pitta energy being responsible for transformation, metabolism, and understanding the senses and emotions.

prakruti—literally means "first action." In Ayurveda it refers to the inherent 'nature' of an individual; their body type and basic mental/emotional state.

purva karma—preliminary procedure to pancha karma, involving warm oil massage and application of heat to initiate the mobilization of toxins trapped in the tissues.

rakta—blood tissue.

rakta moksha—purification of blood using herbs and blood letting.

rasa—plasma.

rasayanas—rejuvenative substances.

rishi—sage of ancient India.

santarpana—mind.

shirobhyanga—head massage.

shirodhara—application of a fine stream of warm oil or milk to the third eye. The oil is sometimes perfumed or medicated.

shukra—male and female reproductive tissues.

siddha taila—massage oil.

srotas—body channel for physical substance of subtle electromagnetic energy.

tapa sweda—dry heat as from a fire, the sun, sauna, or sweat lodge.

tridosha—the three constitutions—vata, pitta, and kapha.

tridoshic—food or phenomena that are balancing to all the constitutions.

triphala—herbal combination of amalaki, bibitaki, and haritaki that improves the elimination of toxins and rejuvenative tissues.

ubtan—paste applied to the body or face and allowed to semi-dry before removing.

ubvartan—vigorously rubbing pastes or powders on the skin.

upadhatu—body tissue that is nourished by a dhatu, but does not nourish any other tissue itself.

upanaha sweda—application of poultices or compresses.

upagni sweda—applications that produce heat in a tissue but are not in themselves hot, i.e. a mustard powder compress.

vamana—therapeutic cleansing of the upper channels using vomiting.

vata—air and ether constitution.

vikruti—imbalance or disorder; may be physical, mental, emotional, or a combination.

virechana—use of a purging laxative to expel waste from the small intestine. Clears excess pitta and kapha dosha.

vyayama—forms of exercise.

yoga—literally means union or joining together. As a general term it means practices that aim to help the individual unite with the universe. Hatha Yoga refers to physical postures that bring strength, flexibility, and poise to the body and peace and clarity to the mind.

SOURCE APPENDIX

To study Ayurvedic medicine:

Ayurvedic Holistic Center
82A Bayville Ave.
Bayville. N.Y. 11709

Ayurvedic Living Workshops
P.O. Box 188
Exeter, Devon EX4 5AB
ENGLAND

The Ayurveda Center of Santa Fe
1807 Second St. Suite 20
Santa Fe, N.M. 87505
(505) 983-8898

Lotus Ayurvedic Center
4145 Clares Street Suite D
Capitola, CA 95010
(408) 479-1667

Maharishi Health Center
Hale Clinic
7 Park Crescent
London, W14 3H3
ENGLAND

Natural Therapeutics Center
'Surya Daya'
Gisingham, Nr. Iye
Suffolk, ENGLAND

Victoria Stern N.D.
P.O. Box 1814
Laguna Beach, CA 92652
(714) 494-8858

Ayurvedic Institute
Dr. Vasant Lad
11311 Menaul NE
Aluquerque, NM 87112
(505) 291-9698

Correspondence courses
American Institute of Vedic Studies
Attn. David Frawley
P.O. Box 8357
Santa Fe, N.M. 87504
(505) 983-9385

Lessons and Lectures in Ayurveda by
Dr. Robert Svoboda
P.O. Box 23445
Albuquerque, N.M. 87192-1445
(505) 291-9698

Institute for Wholistic Education
33719 116th St.
Twin Lakes, WI 53181
Beginner and Advanced Correspondence Courses in Ayurveda

To train in Ayurvedic Facial Massage and Beauty Practices:

Melanie Sachs
"Invoking Beauty with Ayurveda"
Seminars
P.O. Box 13753-3753
San Luis Obispo, CA 93406
(800) 484-6283 ext. 7816

Ayurvedic massage training and yoga therapy:

Margo Gal
1701 Santa Fe River Road
Santa Fe, N.M. 87501
(505) 983-5077

To receive Pancha Karma:

The Ayurveda Center of Santa Fe
1807 Second St. Suite 20
Santa Fe, N.M. 87505
(505) 983-8898

Diamond Way Health Associates
214 Girard Blvd. N.E.
Albuquerque, N.M. 87106
(505) 265-4826

Lotus Ayurvedic Center
4145 Clares Street Suite D
Capitola, CA 95010
(408) 479-1667

Maharishi Health Center
Hale Clinic
7 Park Crescent
London, W14 3H3
ENGLAND

Dr. Lobsang Rapgay
2931 Tilden Ave.
Los Angeles, CA 90064
(310) 477-3877

Victoria Stern N.D.
P.O. Box 1814
Laguna Beach, CA 92652
(714) 494-8858

To get Ayurvedic Herbs and Supplies:

Auroma Int'l.
P.O. Box 1008, Dept. ABC
Silver Lake, WI 53170
(414) 889-8569

Ayush Herbs Inc.
10025 N.E. 4th Street
Bellevue, WA 98004
(800) 925-1371

Bazaar of India Imports, Inc.
1810 University Ave.
Berkeley, CA 94703
(510) 548-4110

Bioveda
P.O. Box 420
Conger, N.Y. 10920

Dr. Singha's Mustard Bath and More
Attn. Anna Searles
Natural Therapeutic Centre
2500 Side Cove
Austin, TX 78704
(800) 856-2862

Herbalvedic Products
P.O. Box 6390
Santa Fe, N.M. 87502

Kanak
P.O. Box 13653
Albuquerque, N.M. 87192-3653

Internatural (retail)
33719 116th St., Dept. ABC
Twin Lakes, WI 53181
(800) 643-4221
www.internatural.com

Lotus Herbs
1505 42nd Ave., Suite 19
Capitola, CA 95010
(408) 479-1667

Lotus Light (wholesale)
P.O. Box 1008, Dept. ABC
Silver Lake, WI 53170
(800) 548-3824

Maharishi Ayurveda Products International Inc.
417 Bolton Road
P.O. Box 541
Lancaster, MA 01523
(for information) 1-800-843-8332 Ext. 903
(to order) 1-800-255-8332 Ext. 903

Yoga of Life Center
2726 Tramway N.E.
Albuquerque, N.M. 87122
(505) 275-6141

Ayurvedic Cosmetic Companies:

Bindi Facial Skin Care
A Division of Pratima Inc.
109-17 72nd Road, Lower Level
Forest Hills, New York 11375
(718) 268-7348

Devi Inc. (for Shivani product line)
P.O. Box 377
Lancaster, Mass. 01523
(attn. Anjali Mahaldar)
(800) 237-8221 FAX (508) 368-0455

Dr. Singha's Mustard Bath and More
Attn. Anna Searles
Natural Therapeutic Centre
2500 Side Cove
Austin, TX 78704
(800) 856-2862

Gajee Herbals
The Khenpo Company
17595 Harvard St. C531
Irvine, CA 92714
(attn. Gayatri Puri, owner)
(714) 250-6027

Herbalvedic Products
P.O. Box 6390
Santa Fe, N.M. 87502
Internatural (retail)
33719 116th St., Dept. ABC
Twin Lakes, WI 53181
(800) 643-4221
www.internatural.com

Lotus Light (wholesale)
P.O. Box 1008, Dept. ABC
Silver Lake, WI 53170
(800) 548-3824

Swami Sada Shiva Tirtha
Ayurvedic Holistic Center
82A Bayville Ave.
Bayville, N.Y. 11709
(phone and fax—(516) 628-8200)

TEJ Beauty Enterprises Inc.
(an Ayurvedic Beauty Salon)
162 West 56th St. Room 201
New York, N.Y. 10019
(owner: Pratima Raichur, founder of Bindi)
(212) 581-8136

Natural Ingredients:

Aloe Farms
Box 125
Los Fresnos, TX 78566
(800) 262-6771
(for aloe vera juice, gel, powder, and
    capsules)

Arya Laya Skin Care Center
Rolling Hills Estates, CA 90274
(for carrot oil)

Aubrey Organics
4419 North Manhattan Ave.
Tampa, FL 33614
(for rosa mosquita oil and a large variety
    of natural cosmeticsand shampoos)

Body Shop
45 Horsehill Road
Cedar Knolls, N.J. 07927-2014
(800) 541-2535
(aloe vera, nut and seed oils, cosmetics,
    make-up, brushes, loofas, and much more)

Culpepper Ltd.
21 Bruton St.
London W1X 7DA
ENGLAND
(variety of natural seed, nut, and kernel
    oils, essential oils, herbs, books, and
    cosmetics)

Desert Whale Jojoba Co.
P.O. Box 41594
Tucson, AZ 85717
(602) 882-4195
(for jojoba products and many other
    natural oils, including rice bran,
    pecan, macadamia nut and apricot
    kernel)

Everybody Ltd.
1738 Pearl St.
Boulder, CO 80302
(800) 748-5675
(large variety of oils, oil blends, and
    cosmetics)

Flora Inc.
P.O. Box 950
805 East Badger Road
Lynden, WA 98264
(800) 446-2110
(for flax seed oil, herbal supplements for
    skin, hair, and nails,and cosmetics

Green Earth Farm
P.O. Box 672
65½ North 8th Street
Saguache, CO 81149
(for calendula oil, creme, and herbal bath)

The Heritage Store Inc.
P.O. Box 444
Virginia Beach, Virginia 23458
(804) 428-0100
(castor oil, organic ghee, cocoa butter,
    massage oils, flowerwaters, essential
    oils, cosmetics, and natural home
    remedies)

Janca's Jojoba Oil and Seed Company
456 E. Juanita #7
Mesa, AZ 85204 (602) 497-9494
(jojoba oil, butter, wax, and seeds. Also a
    large variety of naturally pressed
    unusual oils, such as camellia, kukui
    nut, and grapeseed. Also have clay,
    aloe products. essential oils, and their
    own line of cosmetics)

Internatural (retail)
33719 116th St., Dept. ABC
Twin Lakes, WI 53181
(800) 643-4221
www.internatural.com
Over 8,000 natural body care,
fragrance & herbal products.

Lotus Light (wholesale)
P.O. Box 1008, Dept. ABC
Silver Lake, WI 53170
(800) 548-3824

Weleda Inc.
841 South Main St.
Spring Valley, N.Y. 10977
(for calendula oil and a large variety of
    natural cosmetics)

Aromatherapy Study Programs:

Aromatherapy Video and Home Study
    Program
Michael Scholes (Founder of Aroma Vera)
3384 South Robertson Place
Los Angeles, CA 90034
(800) 677-2368

Jeanne Rose Aromatherapy and Herbal
    Healing Intensives
219 Carl Street
San Francisco, CA 94117
Attn. Jeanne Rose

London School of Aromatherapy
P.O. Box 780
London NW5 1DY
ENGLAND

Pacific Institute of Aromatherapy
P.O. Box 8723
San Rafael, CA 94903
Attn. Kurt Schnaubelt
(515) 479-9121

Quintessence Aromatherapy
P.O. Box 4996
Boulder, CO 80306
Attn. Ann Berwick (303) 258-3791

Essential Oil Supplies:

Aromatherapy Supply
Unit W3
The Knoll Business Center
Old Shoreham Road
Hove, Sussex BN3 7GS
ENGLAND

Aroma Vera
3384 South Robertson Place
Los Angeles, CA 90034
(800) 669-9514

Auroma International, Inc.
P.O. Box 1008, Dept. ABC
Silver Lake, WI 53170
(414) 889-8569
(incense & oils)

Fenmail Tisserand Oils
P.O. Box 48
Spalding, LINCS PE11 ADS
ENGLAND

Lotus Brands
P.O. Box 325, Dept. ABC
Twin Lakes, WI 53181
(414) 889-8561

Internatural (retail)
33719 116th St., Dept. ABC
Twin Lakes, WI 53181
(800) 643-4221
www.internatural.com

Lotus Light (wholesale)
P.O. Box 1008, Dept. ABC
Silver Lake, WI 53170
(800) 548-3824

Private Universe
P.O. Box 3122
Winter Park, Florida 32790
(407) 644-7203

Oshadi Ayus—Quality Life Products
15, Monarch Bay Plaza Suite 346
Monarch Beach, CA 92629
(800) 947-1008 FAX (714) 240-1104

Primavera
D. 8961 Sulzberg
Germany
08376-808-0

Original Swiss Aromatics
P.O. Box 606
San Rafael, CA 94915
(415) 459-3998

Beauty and Quality Ayurvedic Supplements:

Herbalvedic Products
P.O. Box 6390
Santa Fe, N.M. 87502

Internatural (retail)
33719 116th St., Dept. ABC
Twin Lakes, WI 53181
(800) 643-4221
www.internatural.com

Lotus Light (wholesale)
P.O. Box 1008, Dept. ABC
Silver Lake, WI 53170
(800) 548-3824

Maharishi Ayur-Veda Products
    International Inc.
417 Bolton Road
P.O. Box 54
Lancaster, Mass. 01523
(800) ALL-VEDA FAX (508) 368-7475

New Moon Extracts
P.O. Box 1947
Brattleborough, Vermont 05302-1947
(800) 543-7279

Spectrum Natural Omega 3 Oil
The Oil Company
133 Copeland St.
Petaluma, CA 94952

Exercise Programs and Information:

Callanetic Headquarters
1700 Broadway Suite 2000
Denver, CO 80290
(303) 831-4455

Diamond Way Health Associates
214 Girard Blvd. N.E.
Albuquerque, N.M. 87106
(515) 265-4826
(for Sotai, Tibetan Rejuvenation Exercises)

Vega Study Center
1511 Robinson Street
Oroville, CA 95965
(916) 533-7702
(for Sotai instructions—books)

Satori Resources
732 Hamlin Way
San Leandro, CA 94578
(for Tai Chi Chih)

Kushi Institute
P.O. Box 7
Becket, MA 01223
(413) 623-5741
(for Do-in)

Pancha Karma Supplies:

Vicki Stern
P.O. Box 1814
Laguna Beach, CA 92651
(714) 494-8858
(for steam boxes)

Color, Sound, and Gems:

For assessing gems suited to your Vedic
    astrological birthchart:
Dr. David Frawley
1701 Santa Fe River Road
Santa Fe, N.M. 87501
(505) 983-9385

For open-backed gemstone settings:
PAZ
P.O. Box 4859
Albuquerque, N.M. 87196

Color Therapy Eyewear
c/o Terri Perrigone-Messer
P.O. Box 3114
Diamond Springs, CA 95619

Lumatron (light device)
c/o Ernie Baker
515 Pierce St. #3
San Francisco, CA 94117
(415) 626-0083

Internatural (retail)
33719 116th St., Dept. ABC
Twin Lakes, WI 53181
(800) 643-4221
www.internatural.com

Lotus Light (wholesale)
P.O. Box 1008, Dept. ABC
Silver Lake, WI 53170
(800) 548-3824

Genesis (sound device)
Medical Massage Therapy
Attn: Tina Shinn
1857 Northwest Blvd. Annex
Columbus, Ohio 43212
(614) 488-5244

Non-denominational Meditation Training:

Shambhala Training International
Executive Offices
1084 Tower Road
Halifax, Nova Scotia
CANADA B3H 265

Videos:

Feldenkrais Resources
(800) 765-1907

Internatural (retail)
33719 116th St., Dept. ABC
Twin Lakes, WI 53181
(800) 643-4221
www.internatural.com

Wishing Well Video
(wholesale & retail)
P.O. Box 1008, Dept. ABC
Silver Lake, WI 53170
(800) 888-9355

INDEX

Sources of Supply:

The following companies have an extensive selection of useful products and a long track-record of fulfillment. They have natural body care, aromatherapy, flower essences, crystals and tumbled stones, homeopathy, herbal products, vitamins and supplements, videos, books, audio tapes, candles, incense and bulk herbs, teas, massage tools and products and numerous alternative health items across a wide range of categories.

WHOLESALE:

Wholesale suppliers sell to stores and practitioners, not to individual consumers buying for their own personal use. Individual consumers should contact the RETAIL supplier listed below. Wholesale accounts should contact with business name, resale number or practitioner license in order to obtain a wholesale catalog and set up an account.

Lotus Light Enterprises, Inc.

P O Box 1008 ABC
Silver Lake, WI 53170 USA
414 889 8501 (phone)
414 889 8591 (fax)
800 548 3824 (toll free order line)

RETAIL:

Retail suppliers provide products by mail order direct to consumers for their personal use. Stores or practitioners should contact the wholesale supplier listed above.

Internatural

33719 116th Street ABC
Twin Lakes, WI 53181 USA
800 643 4221 (toll free order line)
414 889 8581 office phone
WEB SITE: www.internatural.com

Web site includes an extensive annotated catalog of more than 7000 products that can be ordered "on line" for your convenience 24 hours a day, 7 days a week.